Health-Related Quality of Life - Measurement Tools, Predictors and Modifiers

Edited by Jasneth Mullings, Sage Arbor and Medhane Cumbay

Published in London, United Kingdom

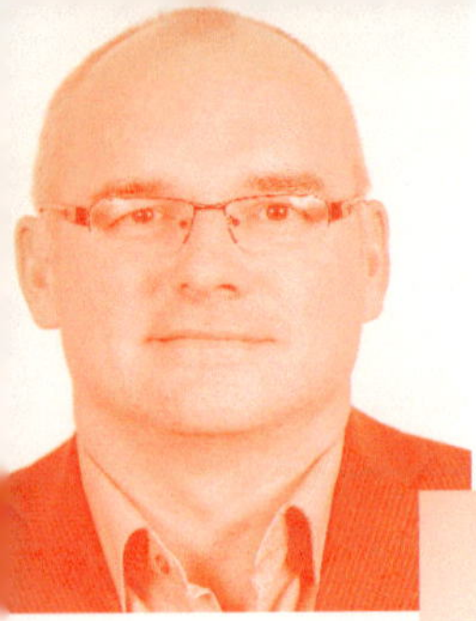
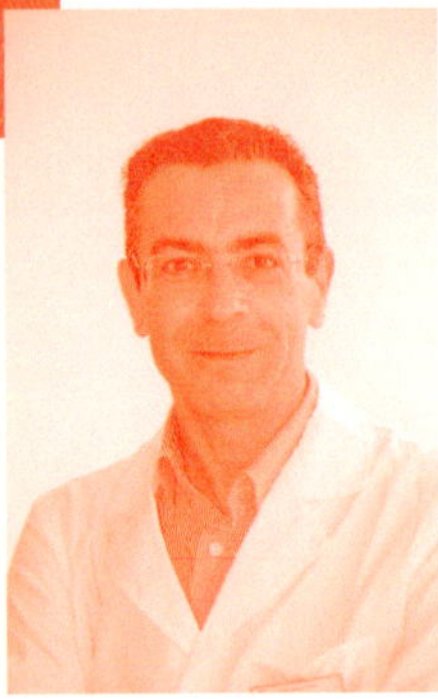
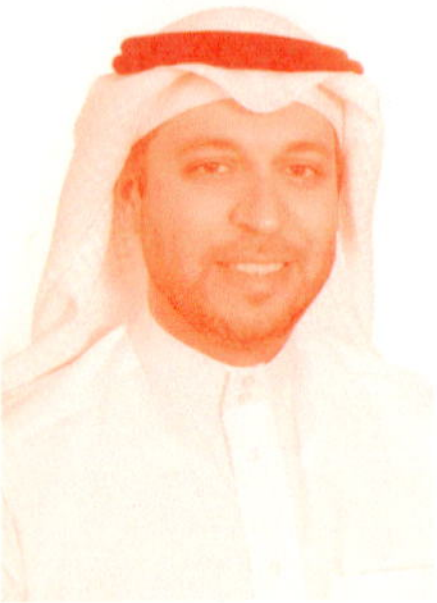
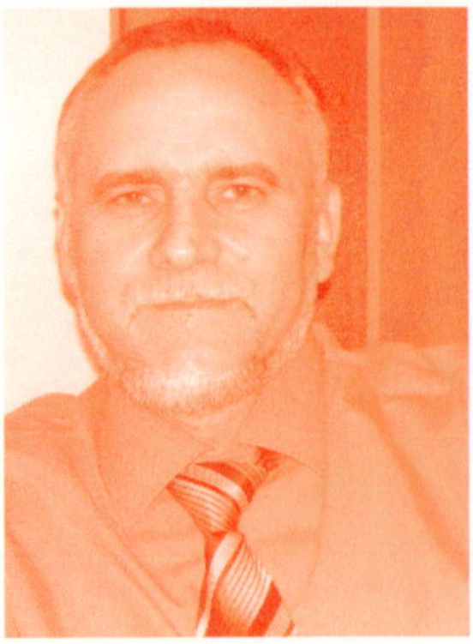
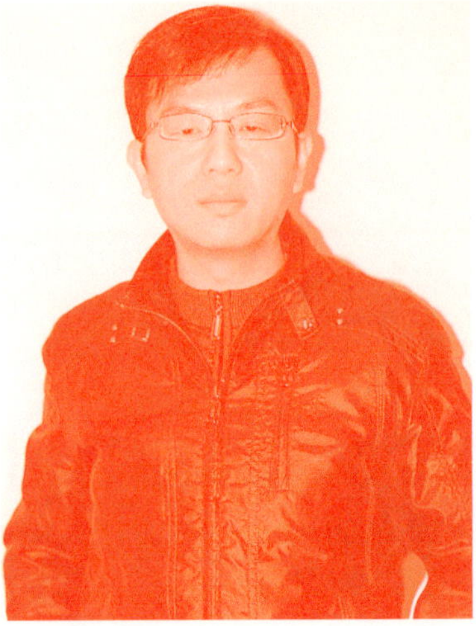
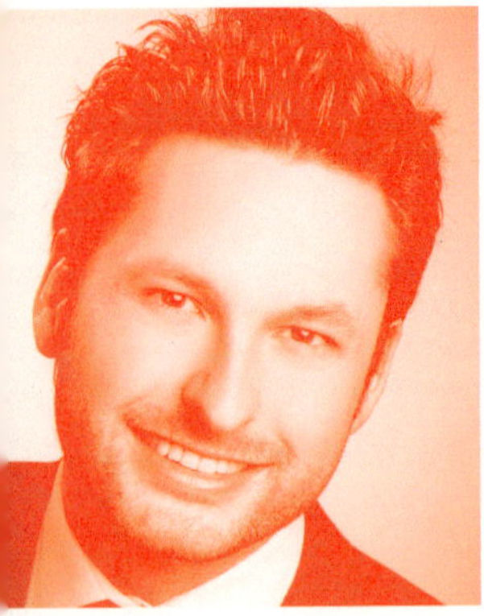
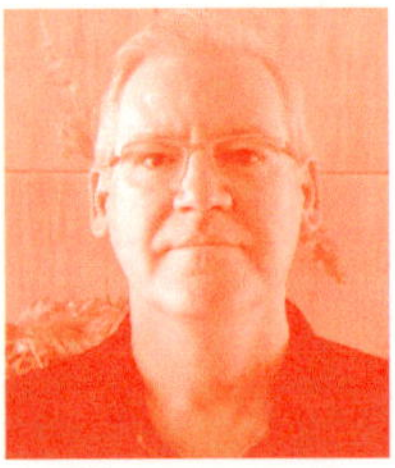

IntechOpen

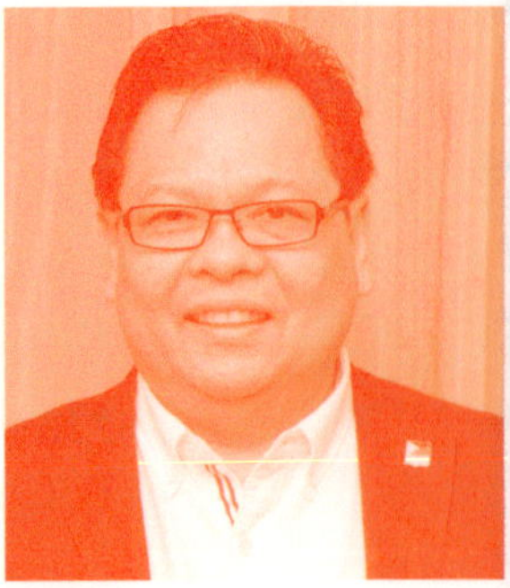
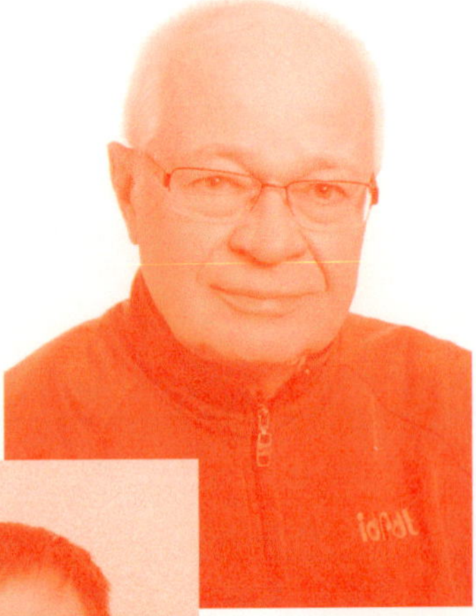
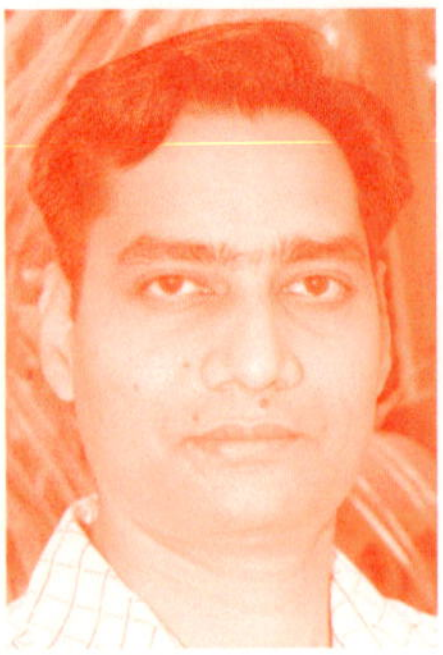
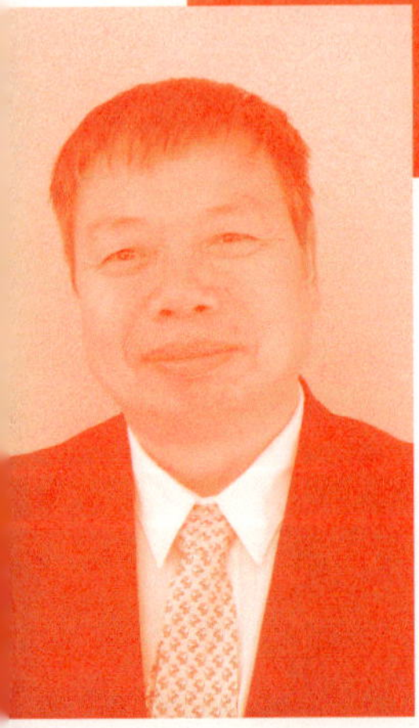
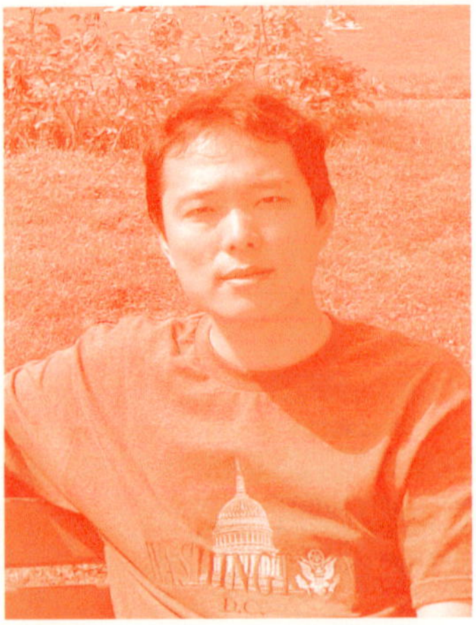
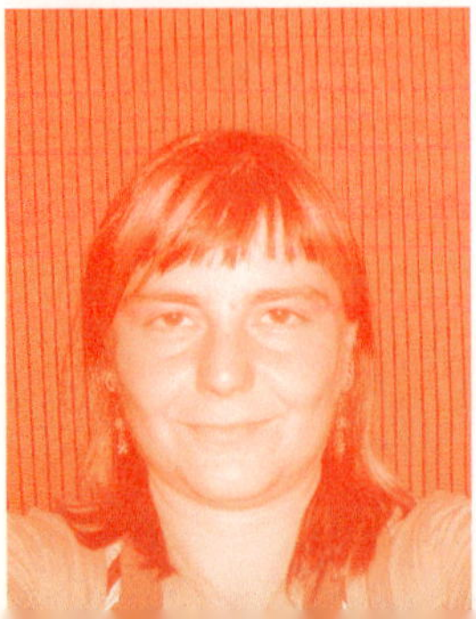

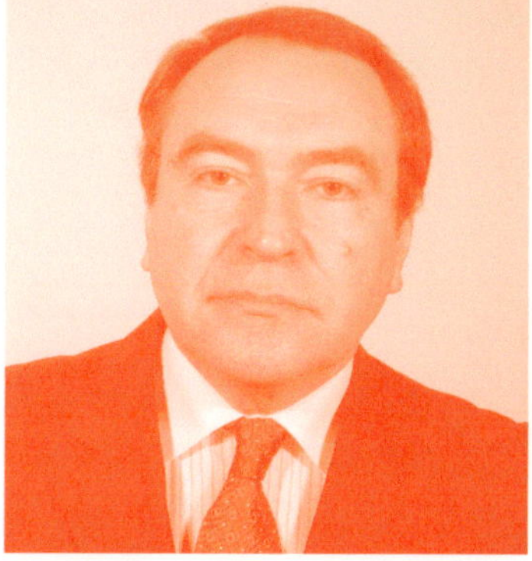
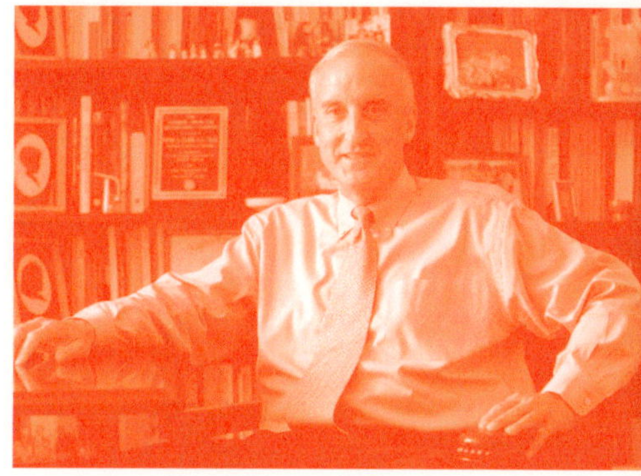
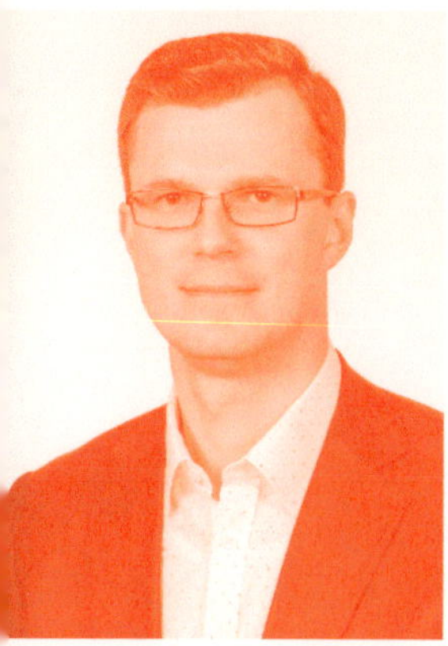
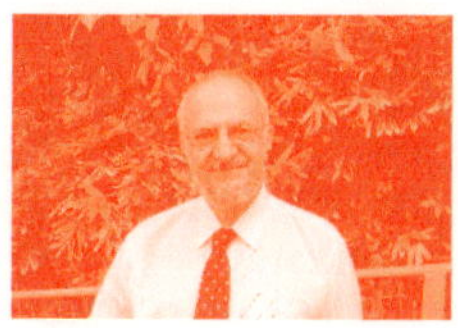
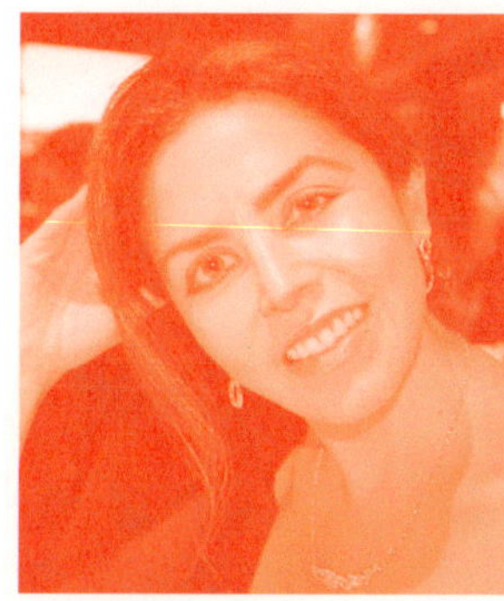

Supporting open minds since 2005

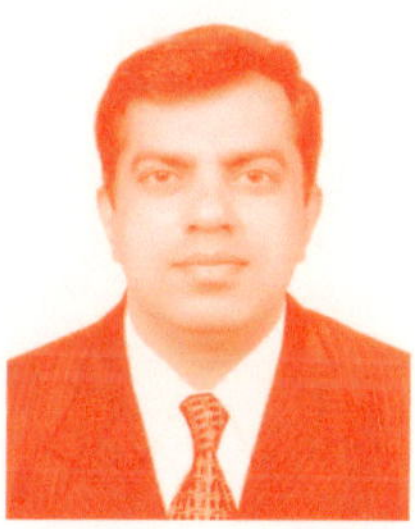
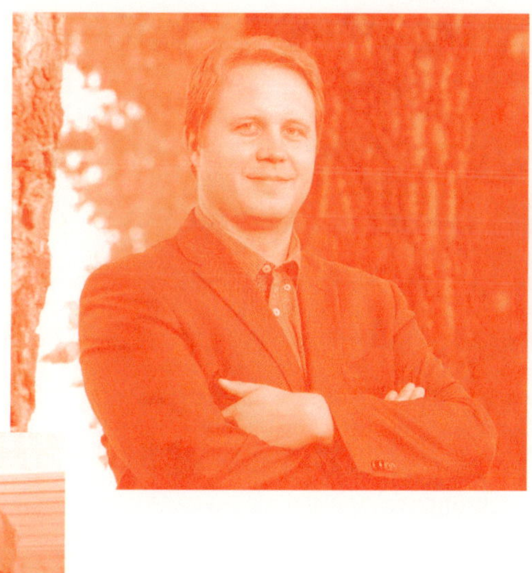
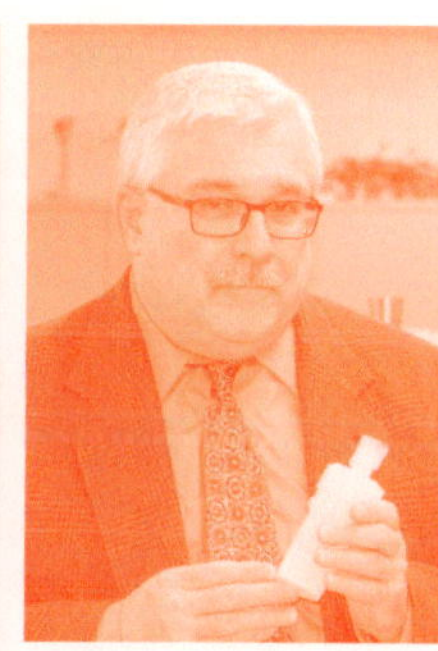
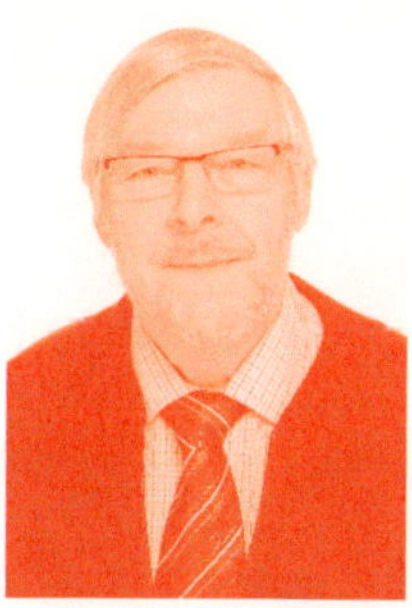
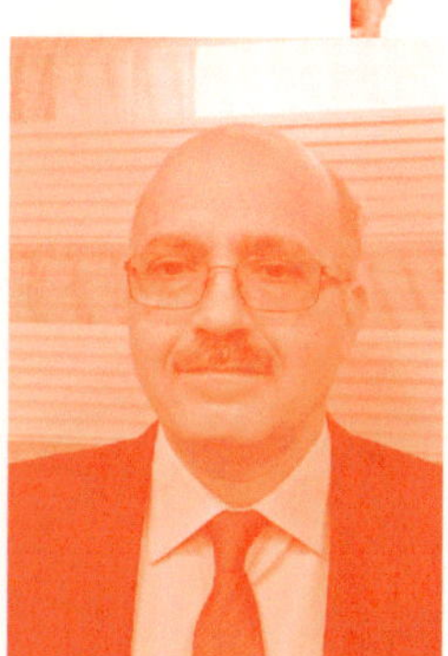
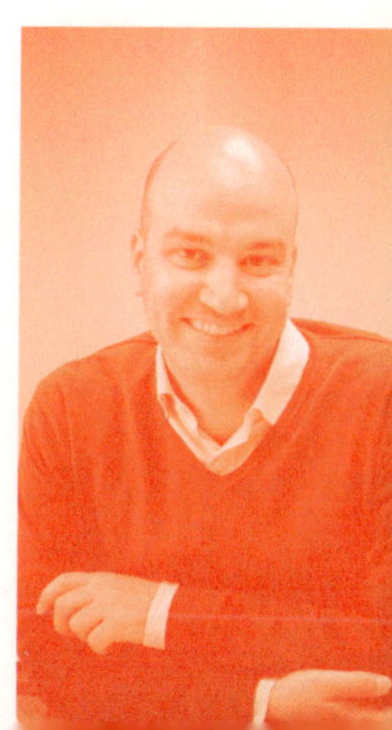
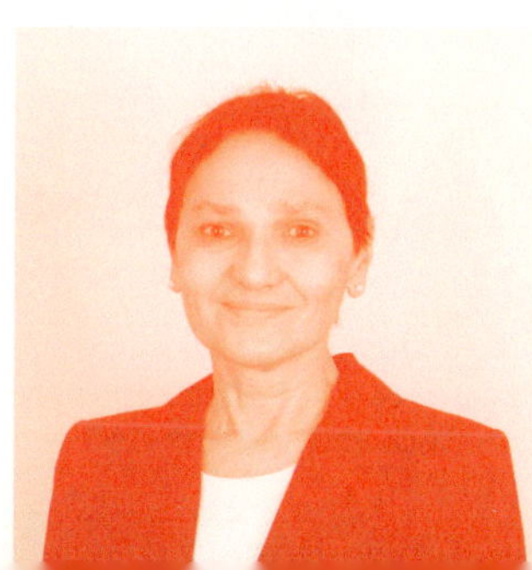

Health-Related Quality of Life - Measurement Tools, Predictors and Modifiers
http://dx.doi.org/10.5772/intechopen.92935
Edited by Jasneth Mullings, Sage Arbor and Medhane Cumbay

Assistant to the Editors: Andrea McPherson, Mona Sue Ho

Contributors
Brendan P. Carmody, Filiz Çömez Polat, Bikila Regassa Feyisa, Trinidad Montero-Vílchez, Salvador Arias-Santiago, Antonio Martinez-López, Manuel Sánchez-Díaz, Margarita del Valle Chacin Fuenmayor, Josymar Chacin de Fernandez, Jose Antonio Miron Canelo, Maria-Fernanda Gómez Lorenzo, Elena Iglesias De Sena, Luz Celia Fernández Martín, Michał Piotr Budzik, Urszula Religioni, Aleksandra Czerw, Andrzej Deptała, Anna M. Badowska-Kozakiewicz, Sage Arbor, Daniela Sacramento Zanini, Larissa de Oliveira e Ferreira, Karina Ferreira Leao Junqueira

First published in London, United Kingdom, 2022 by IntechOpen
IntechOpen is the global imprint of INTECHOPEN LIMITED, registered in England and Wales, registration number: 11086078, 5 Princes Gate Court, London, SW7 2QJ, United Kingdom
Printed in Croatia

British Library Cataloguing-in-Publication Data
A catalogue record for this book is available from the British Library

Additional hard and PDF copies can be obtained from orders@intechopen.com

Health-Related Quality of Life - Measurement Tools, Predictors and Modifiers
Edited by Jasneth Mullings, Sage Arbor and Medhane Cumbay
p. cm.
Print ISBN 978-1-83969-020-4
Online ISBN 978-1-83969-021-1
eBook (PDF) ISBN 978-1-83969-022-8

For EU product safety concerns:
IN TECH d.o.o., Prolaz Marije Krucifikse Kozulić 3, 51000 Rijeka, Croatia, info@intechopen.com or visit our website at intechopen.com.

Meet the editors

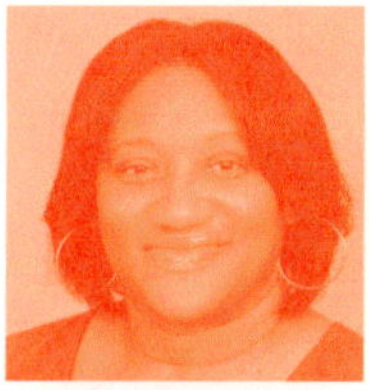

Jasneth Mullings, Ph.D., is a social epidemiologist in the Faculty of Medical Sciences, the University of the West Indies at Mona, Jamaica. Her research focuses on the mental health effects of neighborhood structural and social processes and she serves as a strategic advisor to UrbanHealth360, global thought leaders in urban health.

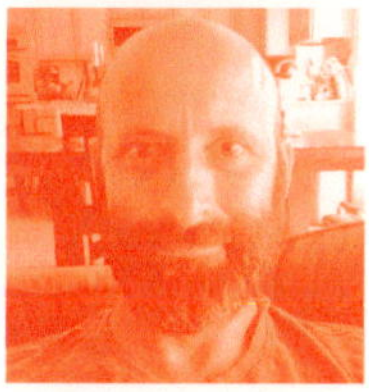

Sage Arbor is a computational biologist whose research includes fields ranging from drug design, systems biology, and epigenetic database creation to fitness app development. His work spans a broad biomedical spectrum from drug design to clinical trial analysis, including being a medical school professor and researcher, project management of developers/analysts of globally distributed labs, electronic medical record data mining (SQL and NoSQL), Python/pandas coding, data segmentation, 6σ improvement, pathway mapping, and computational drug design and synthesis. Having worked at multiple academic institutions (Duke, Marian University) and companies (e.g., Pfizer and Dupont), his research has been on both proprietary and open-access datasets for publication to the wider scientific community. His recent publication topics include quality of life modifiers, therapeutic interventions for Alzheimer's disease, bioethical versus religious standards, and scientific training in those deciding public policy.

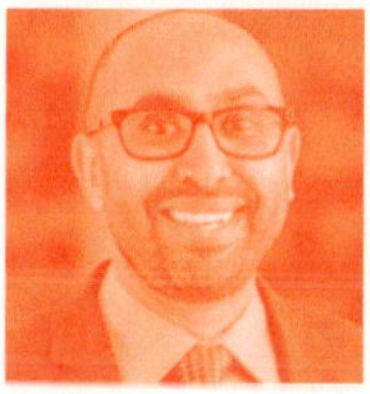

Dr. Medhane Cumbay has extensive experience in cell surface receptor function as it relates to cellular signaling, elucidating drug-receptor interactions, neurodegenerative diseases, and drug development. He earned a BS in Biochemistry and Biophysics from Oregon State University in 1995. While working with multiple research groups at Oregon Health Sciences University between 1995 and 1998, Dr. Cumbay developed an interest in neuroscience and neuropharmacology. This led him to pursue a doctoral degree at Purdue University, Indiana, where he earned a Ph.D. in Molecular Pharmacology in 2004. He completed a postdoctoral fellowship at the Stark Neuroscience Research Institute, Indiana University School of Medicine. He joined the faculty at Butler University, Indiana, in 2007, and the Marian University College of Osteopathic Medicine, Indiana, in 2015.

Contents

Preface

Quality of life (QoL) is an important construct for health and wellbeing, with applications for clinical care, research, and individual or patient use. An assessment of QoL acknowledges the significance of modifiable and non-modifiable risk factors for health and disease (1, 2). QoL also has broader implications as a social and developmental concept. As defined by the World Health Organization (WHO), quality of life is "individuals' perceptions of their position in life in the context of the culture and value systems in which they live and in relation to their goals, expectations, standards, and concerns" (3). This definition takes cognizance of the subjective nature of QoL, and its immersion in the context of societal, cultural, and environmental norms.

With growing interest in QoL and the development of more comprehensive approaches to measurement, numerous methodologies and tools have been developed to measure Health-Related Quality of Life (HRQoL) and associated domains. The World Health Organization Quality of Life (WHOQOL) assessment measures this "multi-dimensional concept, incorporating the individual's perception of health status, psycho-social status and other aspects of life" (4). The WHOQOL-100 tool is a cross-cultural instrument that measures domains of physical, psychological, social relationships, environment, and spirituality/religion/personal beliefs (4).

Section 1 of this book, "Quality of Life Indicators and Measurements," introduces the concepts of health-related quality of life (HRQoL) and the measures used in its assessment. Chapter 1, "Modifiers of Health-Related Quality of Life by Biological, Psychological and Social Factors" by Canelo, Lorenzo Gómez, De Sena, and Fernández-Martín, establishes the concept of HRQoL, reviews frequently used tools, and makes recommendations for their application in clinical care. This chapter offers a guide for clinicians, public health practitioners, and researchers.

Quality-adjusted life years (QALYs) measures years of life, adjusted for the QoL during those years. It serves as a measure of longevity and health outcomes (5). In Chapter 2, "Ethical Issues which Have Prevented the U.S. from Maximizing Quality of Life Years", the author Sage Arbor argues the value of QALYs for resource allocation and discusses the societal norms that challenge its effective utilization. The author highlights forces such as age, sex, lifestyle (e.g., smoking, drinking, obesity), cost transparency, and societal and demographic transitions (e.g., war, population explosion vs. collapse) that present ethical dilemmas for the use of QALYs.

Section 2, "Assessing Quality of Life in States of Chronic Diseases and Psychological Health," addresses HRQoL in the context of chronic diseases, including psychological dimensions and interventions. Chapter 3, "Assessment of Pain, Acceptance of Illness, Adjustment to Life and Strategies of Coping with the Illness in Patients with Pancreatic Cancer" by Religioni, Czerw, Badowska-Kozakiewicz, Budzik, and Deptała, reports on coping strategies and life adjustments for a sample of patients living with pancreatic cancer, the fourth most common type of cancer worldwide. In Chapter 4, "Predictors of Health-Related Quality of Life among Patients with

Diabetes Mellitus," Regassa Feyisa makes the for the need to measure HRQol for persons living with diabetes in Ethiopia. In this chapter, predictors of HRQoL were identified as age, sex, marital status, educational status, feelings of being stigmatized, co-morbidity status, chronic complication, and body mass index. In Chapter 5, "Quality of Life in Patients with Skin Disease and Their Cohabitants" by Montero-Vílchez, Sánchez-Díaz, Martínez-López, and Arias-Santiago, documents the significant impact of chronic skin diseases on QoL for both those directly and indirectly affected by skin conditions. The authors present a literature review of the psychological and social impact on both groups.

In Chapter 6, "Psychological Intervention Based on Psychoneuroimmunology in Children and Adult," Margarita del Valle Chacin Fuenmayor and Josymar Chacin de Fernandez describe the evolution of psychoneuroimmunology (PNI). This emerging field of study examines the contribution of the mind to the development of disease as well as prevention and treatment. The authors discuss the influence of stress on health and the role of PNI in managing disease and improving quality of life.

Section 3 presents "Quality of Life in the Context of the Social Gradient and Social Determinants of Health." Social factors are critical in the health determinants matrix and are shaped by economics, social policies, and politics. Undoubtedly, social resources influence QoL, significantly impacting population health outcomes. The evidence shows that health inequities are driven by social determinants, such as access to education, housing, income levels, and public safety (6). Furthermore, the concept of the social gradient where life expectancy is lower further down the social ladder is key to understanding the impact of poverty on health and QoL (7). Violence and exposure to the same is a byproduct of socioeconomic, cultural, and political forces and directly influences HRQoL. Globally, violence is recognized and treated as a public health problem and approaches to address it have largely been through the public health lens of identifying the causes and correlates, developing intervention interventions and public education programmes (8). An important aspect is a structural violence, which are those injustices embedded within social and institutional structures, which have been shown to drive health inequalities (9, 10), for example, disparities in education, income, and access to health and social resources (11, 12, 13) . Filiz Çömez Polat discusses the relationship between poverty and psychological processes in Chapter 7, "Poverty and Social Psychology: The Importance of Integrative Manner." The author argues the role of the empirical study of the social-psychological correlates of poverty in making a salient contribution to poverty reduction. In Chapter 8, "Zambia's Poorest Progressively Left Behind: Well-Being Denied," Brendan Carmody chronicles the history of the post-independence efforts of the Zambian government, which were aimed at revolutionizing the education system to secure greater equity, prosperity, and inclusiveness for the population. The chapter presents the challenges and deficiencies of the process, which the author argues has unfortunately opened the door to the marginalization of the majority.

The concluding chapter by Zanini Daniela, et al. "Living with Violence and its Relationship with Executive Function (EF) in Childhood and Adolescence: Literature Review," reviews the literature on the relationship between violence and the development of executive function in children and adolescents. The authors asserts that the evidence indicates that living with violence impairs the nuclear components of EF (i.e., working memory, cognitive flexibility, and inhibitory control) and makes the case for further research and public policy investments to stem the tide of violence.

QoL assessments provide important tools for the quantitative and qualitative measurement of wellbeing and health outcomes. This book shares a global experience of QoL measures across various disease states and social environments, integrating developed and developing world reports. The findings shared by authors from across the globe may be informative for patients, healthcare providers, researchers, and policymakers alike.

The editors acknowledge the significant support of assistants to the editor Andrea Norman-McPherson of the University of the West Indies (UWI) School of Nursing, Mona at the UWI, and Mona J. Sue-Ho of the Jamaica Social Investment Fund in the completion of this work.

Jasneth Mullings
Faculty of Medical Sciences,
The University of the West Indies,
Mona Kingston, Jamaica

Sage Arbor and Medhane Cumbay
Marian University,
Indiana, United States of America

Tomlin Paul
University of the West Indies,
Kingston, Jamaica

Section 1

Quality of Life Indicators and Measurements

Chapter 1

Modifiers of Health-Related Quality of Life by Biological, Psychological and Social Factors

Jose Antonio Miron Canelo, Maria-Fernanda Lorenzo Gómez, Elena Iglesias De Sena and Luz Celia Fernández Martín

Abstract

Healthcare workers, clinicians and/or researchers require information on the consequences of illness on their patients, as well as on the effects associated with treatments, when making decisions on recommended treatments and for follow-up evaluations of the same. Identifying health indicators which provide necessary and appropriate data for the evaluation of clinical outcomes in terms of Health-Related Quality of Life (HRQoL), as established by the WHO Biopsychosocial Model, and which provide appropriate and pertinent information on physical, mental and social factors in patients, can improve decision-making in relation to a comprehensive and global perspective of clinical outcomes of the various treatments and procedures given to patients. This chapter aims to provide an overview of the various tools for assessing Health-Related Quality of Life, as a growing number of clinicians, researchers and patient groups wish for comprehensive and not merely biological measures of health. This may be explained by the growing number of self-administered or interview questionnaires which have the aim of measuring changes in health as well as the consequences of the various treatments used mainly on chronicity and chronic health conditions. During recent decades, numerous tools have been developed and applied to the measurement of the effects of Health-Related Quality of Life in patients based on biological or physical aspects, psychological or mental aspects, and social aspects. This chapter will review the most frequently-used tools for the measurement of Health-Related Quality of Life, and recommendations are made for their use in medical care according to psychometric characteristics and quality criteria, as a guide for use in the field of healthcare, in public health, or in outcomes research.

Keywords: Health-Related Quality of Life (HRQoL), health conditions, medical care

1. Introduction

The term "health indicator" refers to a characteristic associated to the health of an individual or a population. In Public Health and in Health Planning, population health indicators are used to show the magnitude of a medical problem, to reflect a change in the health status of a patient or a population over time, to compare and assess differences in health status among patients and populations, and to analyse and evaluate the extent to which treatment goals have been achieved in patients in order to recommend these treatments for use in clinical practice and research [1, 2].

Measurement of health and Health-Related Quality of Life (HRQoL) has acquired great importance in recent decades as a means of measuring clinical outcomes in patients and of monitoring the progress of various treatments along with their physical, psychological and social consequences [3]. Medical practitioners frequently must choose from among diverse tools with the aim of obtaining essential relevant information for decisions on treatment, with analysis and a multidimensional assessment of these treatments on patients.

Meanwhile, countries have health information systems which permit the development of a wide variety of health indicators, and thus allow periodic surveys of their healthcare situation. These indicators provide information on their change over time, which makes it possible to assess trends and geographical distributions. Likewise, the wide availability of these indicators allows comparison with other countries [4, 5].

Selection of indicator sets is commonly done in countries with well-developed health information systems with the aim of providing executive and multidimensional information. Among global health indicators are those whose objective is to assess the perception of improvement in patient functional capacity on a global scale, i.e. assessing subjective patient perception of the physical, mental and social components in a global and comprehensive fashion [6].

The concept of Quality of Life has undergone such rapid development that it is used very frequently and to such an extent that it has become a common expression in both professional settings and the general population. The healthcare sector is not immune to its influence and many professionals rely on it to assess the patient's psychosocial experience and the effects on the disease of medical and surgical interventions and procedures. This term originated in the USA after the end of World War II, during the development of the Welfare State.

The development of HRQoL research is linked to changes during recent decades in the concept of health, whose basis has shifted from a *biomedical* model to a *biopsychosocial* model [7]. This indicator began to be used extensively from the 1980s, especially in connection with the care of chronically ill patients. Patient health and ability to function depends on and is a consequence of several components: physical, mental and social. Therefore patients must be assessed globally and, consequently, the functioning of all three components must be taken into account for a patient to progress as a person and a social individual.

In this context, HRQoL estimates and measures living conditions of patients which are linked to health conditions and/or disease, and has become a fundamental *dependent or response variable* when assessing success of therapeutic or surgical aims in the medical field. In other words, the HRQoL indicator is currently a valuable tool for understanding circumstances linked to disease and medical care.

The first model or framework which was established to measure Quality of Care was described and proposed by *A. Donabedian* [8]. This author proposed a framework, now classic, which evaluates three components. Firstly, ***structure,*** the stable attributes required for care, i.e. the available resources: human, material, technological, financial, etc. This component has been used to accredit hospitals and health centres for teacher training, and to classify hospitals. Teaching posts which are made available for training resident interns are allotted based on this element of quality of care. Secondly, the model must assess and analyse the ***process,*** the actions taken with the available resources; i.e. the use healthcare providers make of what they have in their clinics, clinical services, medico-surgical services, etc. Thirdly,

Quality of Care*	*Structure*	*Process*	*Outcome*
Focus	*What we have*	*What we do*	*What we get*
Measures/Indicators	*Resources*	*Actions*	*Health Status* *HRQoL* *Wellbeing*

**Framework from Avedis Donabedian.*

Table 1.
Classical model of quality of care.

the model considers ***outcome***, i.e. the results in terms of improved health, lifestyle, quality of life and wellbeing (**Table 1**).

The **overall aim** of this chapter is to present the tools for measuring Health-Related Quality of Life (HRQoL) which allow a global, subjective evaluation of patients in connection to the various medical and or surgical procedures which they undergo. These tools should also provide the ability to follow up on the effects and consequences on patients of these procedures from a multidimensional perspective. The information obtained from these indicators enables professional decision-making based on relevant, personal and holistic information about patients. The goal of this chapter is also eminently practical: without entering into theoretical considerations, it will perform a methodological review of these tools to facilitate decision-making when choosing generic and/or specific surveys.

2. Methodology

In the field of health, HRQoL measurements are widely used, to the extent that specialist journals exist while non-specialist journals have also, in recent years, published editorials and articles on the subject. Available information on tools for the measurement of HRQoL has been subjected to a review process according to the following criteria: 1. - Adaptation to the objective. 2.-Psychometric criteria of *validity, reliability* and *discriminative power or sensitivity to change*. 3.- Practical utility for health workers, teachers and researchers in various settings and population groups, such as the general population or vulnerable groups (e.g. chronic patients, individuals with disabilities and dependent or frail persons). The measurement tools included in this chapter were chosen according to whether the questionnaires contain items which evaluate physical, psychological and social factors according to the biopsychosocial health model, which was proposed in the 1970s and adapted by the WHO [7] as a means of evaluating HRQoL and wellbeing in patients and across population groups [9–14]. And these have been selected based on metrical quality criteria of previously selected instruments such as:

2.1 Validity

In the measurement of HRQoL, no single method for assessing the validity of measuring instruments exists, as it is an indirect assessment through indicator systems. In other words, there is no single way for a tool to measure what it is intended to measure through *content validity* based on the analysis of the concept to be measured and with a definition of the dimensions covered such that the indicators represent the dimensions of health status to be analysed and evaluated. *Construct validity,* on the other hand, is the relationship between the variable to be measured and the concept indicator being measured, i.e. health [15–19].

2.2 Reliability

The reliability of an instrument is given by its stability or consistency in observations when the process of measurement is repeated under equal or similar conditions. Several types of reliability may be derived from this definition: *test–retest* (stability of the tool if measurement conditions and concept are unchanged), *interobserver* (if measurement is carried out by multiple observers and the concordance index, kappa, is between 0.8 and 1 [20]), and *internal consistency* (stability of scores among the various elements of the measuring tool) [21].

2.3 Discriminatory power or sensitivity to change

This property requires that small clinical variations due to a treatment or procedure are reflected in the scores given by patients. Evaluating this property is essential in instruments whose sole purpose is assessment. When a measuring tool is used to categorise patients with differing degrees of severity or disability, discriminatory power is vital. A recent study analysed and assessed the Nottingham Health Profile (NHP), the Short Form-36 (SF-36) survey, the Psychological General Well-Being Index (PGWB) and a single-item 0 to 100 Self-Rated Health Scale, evaluating psychometric properties such as internal consistency, construct validity and discriminatory power. The authors conclude that there is high concordance among the three HRQoL tools (PGWB, SF-36 and NHP) in all aspects but the social, and that these tools may identify the presence of self-assessed poor health. The quick, simple Self-Rated Health Scale was strongly correlated with the more time-consuming PGWB, SF-36 and NHP [21]. Reviews have also been published on tools for assessing the properties of instruments measuring quality of life [22].

2.4 Internal consistency

In questionnaires developed to measure different dimensions separately, as it happens when HRQoL is measured, each dimension's internal consistency must be evaluated using Cronbach's alpha. Its values range between 0 and 1 and indicate the degree of agreement between two quantitative variables, similar to the correlation coefficient.

2.5 Strength of recommendation

Following the above psychometric criteria and a qualitative SWOT analysis we identify those tools which meet the criteria of consistency, validity, and discriminative power and which have more strengths than weaknesses and, therefore, represent an opportunity for improving patient HRQoL. While the aim is to provide a quick, eminently practical guide for use in research on health and quality of life for instructors, health workers and researchers, tools must be adapted to socio-clinical context and to specific patients.

In summary, generic measures of quality of life are proposed, contrasted against previous studies and other tools with clinical utility in highly prevalent diseases due to their importance and significance in both the general population and in vulnerable groups (such as elderly individuals with morbidity and multiple pathologies, and disabled and/or dependent individuals).

All these tools seek to convert Evidence-Based Medicine (EBM) into Results-Based Medicine (RBM), taking into account biological, physical, mental, emotional and social components in order to improve patient HRQoL and wellbeing. This evolution from EBM to RBM is very important for chronic patients, elderly individuals, and individuals with disabilities, because those components which provide satisfaction in life are improved and thus improve quality of life and wellbeing.

3. Generic HRQoL tools

3.1 SF-36 survey

One of the best-known and most widely used tools for the measurement of HRQoL internationally is the **SF-36 Survey** [23, 24]. This was developed in the US in the 1990s for use in analysis and assessment of clinical outcomes, based on questionnaires which included a variety of concepts related to health.

This tool consists of 36 questions, 35 of which assess health through eight dimensions covering two areas, Functional Status and Emotional Wellbeing. The functional area is represented by the following dimensions: Physical Function (10 items), Social Function (2 items), Role Limitations due to physical problems (4 items), Role Limitations due to emotional problems (3 items). Wellbeing includes the following dimensions: Mental Health (5 items), Vitality (4 items), Pain (2 items). Finally, overall assessment of health includes the dimension Perception of General Health (5 items) and Change in Health Status over time (1 item). Two versions exist: standard, with a 4-week recall period, and acute, with a 1-week recall period. The 36th question covers perceived changes in health in the year prior to the interview.

The SF-36 survey has good validity, reliability and sensitivity to change, giving this tool a Grade A recommendation, i.e. the survey meets sufficient quality criteria. Experts and practitioners who have employed the survey quote numerous reasons for its use, such as ease of use and interpretation, multidimensional assessment, comparability, and use in vulnerable groups [11–13]. Furthermore, the Short-Form survey has several versions according to number of items (36, 12, 8 or 6), enabling it to be generalised and used in multiple contexts and with diverse aims [25–27]. SF-12 was the most used for assessment of clinical outcomes. These diverse versions show good psychometric properties across different patients, population groups and countries. Therefore SF-36 is shown as an effective and reliable tool for the measurement of clinical outcomes in patients with various conditions and across various population groups such as persons with intellectual disabilities [11, 13]. It has been validated in numerous countries and therefore allows comparisons among patients with diverse health conditions, diseases and medical treatments, as well as comparison with a general reference population. **Table 2** shows the number of items for each component assessed by the survey. These items register both positive and negative changes in health (**Table 2**).

In a review of the survey's measuring ability, reliability, validity and responsiveness to instrument change, conducted on 17 chosen articles which assessed the psychometric characteristics of the questionnaire, the reliability of SF-36 scales was greater than the suggested standard (Cronbach's alpha) of 0.7 in 96% of evaluations. The pooled evaluations obtained by meta-analysis were higher than 0.7 in all cases. SF-36 showed good differentiation among groups of varying severity, moderate correlation with clinical indicators, and high correlation with other HRQoL instruments. In addition, the survey scores predict mortality. Therefore, SF-36 and its derivatives are an appropriate tool for use in medical research, as well as in clinical practice; in some countries attempts were made to add the survey to medical records, though this has been less successful [28].

Consequently, the SF-36 survey is a complete instrument which allows the assessment of generic HRQoL or health status in patients by analysing and

Aspects	Number of items
Physical Functioning	10
Role Limitations: Physical Problems	4
Pain	2
General Health Perceptions	5
Change in Health over Time	1
Vitality	4
Social Functioning	2
Mental Health	5
Role Limitations: Emotional Problems	3

Table 2.
Number of items for each component assessed by the survey.

evaluating various aspects of the patients, and its clinical use is recommended in order to assess the outcomes of treatment or care based on the opinion of the patients, as a reliable, valid tool with sensitivity to change.

Above all, its use is recommended when cure and/or prognosis rates of two treatments are equal, but differences may be seen in the vital and social implications of each treatment (such as chemotherapy with profound side effects, in cases of cancer) or when limitations occur in the patient's life and wellbeing. It may also be used to assess patient satisfaction with the service provided and to assess reintegration to normal life in cases of disabling diseases and conditions or in persons with disabilities [11, 13]. In addition, the survey may be self-administered by patients or be given by an interviewer. According to experts [29], this tool has a Grade A recommendation for its psychometric criteria, for its generalisability for comparisons, and for its recent use in various cohorts such as the elderly and persons with Alzheimer's disease [11–13, 30–32], and in very diverse conditions and circumstances [33–40]. It can therefore be used to assess HRQoL of patients in general and of vulnerable population groups, alone or in combination with other tools. In summary, the SF-36 is a reproducible, short, valid and versatile survey which has even been proposed for use in economic measures of health [41].

3.2 Nottingham health profile

The Nottingham Health Profile was developed in the UK in the late 1970s with the aim of measuring the subjective perception of the impact of health problems. The authors state that it is appropriate for use in assessing medical and/or social interventions, in pre-post or quasi-experimental designs, as a measure of comparisons among cohorts, as a survey tool on selected populations, for long-term follow-up in patients with chronic disease, as a complement to medical history, and for clinical research in selected patient cohorts. In summary, experts state that it is most suitable for patients with significantly impaired health status, because the survey has the *weakness* of lacking items that track positive health [29].

It is a generic tool for measuring the *degree of physical, psychological and social suffering* associated with medical, social and emotional problems that affect the lives of patients.

The survey consists of two parts. The first has 38 questions with 6 dimensions: Energy (3 items), Pain (8 items), Physical Mobility (8 items), Emotional Reactions

(9 items), Sleep (5 items) and Social Isolation (5 items). These items aim to represent various states of health and record Yes/No responses from the patient. The second part consists of 7 questions on health-related limitations to 7 functional activities of daily living: paid employment, household chores, social life, family life, sex life, hobbies and interests, and free or leisure time. The score ranges from 0 to 100 depending on whether a patient's responses are all negative (0) or all positive (100) [42–44]. Six different scores are obtained for each of the dimensions, giving an estimated observation of the patient's perception of their state of health which may be used without staging of the items, simply by taking the number of positive responses divided by the number of items in that dimension and multiplied by 100 to obtain a range of results from 1 to 100 with the same interpretation as globally. The authors recommend the use of scores by dimension, rather than global scores. A short or reduced version exists, with 22 items. It may be self-administered (preferable) or with an interviewer or interviewers. It has been used in patients with coronary disease, lung cancer, undergoing addiction treatment with methadone, and fibromyalgia [45–48]. It is Grade A recommendation for its psychometric criteria, its generalisability for use in comparisons, and for utility in patient follow-up and in diverse conditions and patient cohorts.

3.3 Sickness impact profile (SIP)

The Sickness Impact Profile (SIP) was developed in the United States with the aim of providing a valid and sensitive measure of perceived health status in order to correctly appraise clinical outcomes during evaluation, planning and programming of health policies. It was designed for the assessment and measurement of dysfunction from in types and degrees of severity of patients and their conditions, although it is specifically designed for patients with moderate or severe deficiencies and dysfunctions [29]. The overall objective of the SIP is the measurement of *dysfunction caused by disease* in critical patients [49] and the assessment of quality of life in patients in need of surgical intervention for urinary diversions [50], defining "dysfunction" as an alteration in the manner of approaching and performing any given activity, with total cessation of the same or with total replacement by a novel activity. In other words, it is a useful tool for the evaluation of disability in the field of Occupational Health, which can improve the objectivity of the committees that assess disability and functional impairment. SIP also evaluates capability in activities of daily living such as resting, eating, household management, recreation, walking, personal hygiene and grooming, work, social integration, state of mind, emotional behaviour and ability to communicate [29].

The SIP is based on the patient's perception of their own illness and not on the professional and scientific concept of that illness. This instrument is based around changes in behaviour and activities of daily living (ADLs) as a result of negative effects of diseases and their consequences, on a simple generic HRQoL scale composed of 136 questions grouped into 12 categories. Of these twelve categories, seven can be grouped into two, Physical or Psychosocial, and five are independent. The physical dimension consists of mobility, ambulation, and body care and movement; the psychosocial dimension has four categories: social relationships, intellectual activity, emotional activity and communication. The five independent categories are sleep and rest, eating, hobbies and entertainment, work, and household tasks.

In this tool the patient must mark only the questions which describe their *circumstances and state of health* at the present moment, and those which are related and/or associated with the disease and its consequences. The result ranges from 0 to 100, where 0 is absence of dysfunction and 100 is maximum dysfunction. It is obtained by summing the scalar values of items marked by patients divided by the sum of scalar values of all the SIP items and multiplying by 100. It may be self-administered, which is preferable, or given by an interviewer. It is Grade A for its psychometric criteria [29, 51], for its generalisability for comparisons, and for utility in assessments of patient perception of their own health status and the consequences of various diseases such as incontinence, chronic pain and periodontal disease [52–55].

4. HRQoL indicators for prevalent diseases and functional disability

Measurement tools for health and HRQoL in the field of disease have developed considerably and are generally associated with the most prevalent problems present in the population, and therefore in those with most patients. Among these the following can be highlighted:

4.1 Quality of life profile for the chronically ill (PECVEC)

This standardised tool of measurement was developed in 1996 to assess somatic, emotional and social components as well as functioning and well-being in clinical practice [29, 56]. Therefore it may be used in diverse risk groups and when assessing therapeutic measures and analysing the progression of chronicity. It is composed of 40 questions with a Likert-type response scale with 5 scores, from nothing to a great deal. It is a multidimensional assessment involving the following aspects: Physical Capacity (8 items), Psychological Functioning (8 items), Positive Mood (5 items), Negative Mood (8 items), Social Functioning (6 items) and Social Welfare (5 items). Range of scores is 0 to 4 in all items and the highest score corresponds to the highest quality of life in the patient, with the same weight given to physical and psychological aspects and differentiating between social functioning and social well-being. It has been used successfully in epidemiological studies in the general population and in patients with various chronic diseases such as hypertension, DM, rheumatic disease and acute myocardial infarction. It can be self-administered (preferable) or by an interviewer or interviewers in patients with difficulties, such as persons with visual or intellectual disabilities. It is Grade A for its psychometric criteria, generalisability for comparisons, and utility in assessments of patient perception of their own health status and the consequences of diseases and circumstances on patient quality of life.

4.2 EUROQOL-5D

EQ-5D is a measure of self-perceived health which originated with the desire of integrating the five dimensions considered most relevant to HRQoL: mobility, self-care, habitual activates, pain/discomfort, and anxiety/depression [57]. It is a generic, standardised, self-administered questionnaire, easy to answer and with low cognitive and intellectual load. EQ-5D is widely used around the world, and is available in more than 170 languages, including several versions in Spanish after a rigorous translation process [58, 59]. It is available in multiple formats: paper and electronic. According to the author, EQ-5D's potential in Spain, not merely as a measure of health but also as a basis for economic assessment, would increase if it were systematically incorporated into clinical information [60, 61] and primary care, and were validated for patients with constipation [62]. This can only occur if healthcare professionals consider that patient-submitted information on HRQoL outcomes is relevant to the management of their clinical work. EuroQol was developed with the aim of making a generic instrument for measuring HRQoL which could be used in applied, clinical and public health research, and which allowed comparisons among countries, but which was also capable of detecting and quantifying changes in health status and quality of life. The test was designed to obtain and provide descriptive information on quality of life based on various dimensions, a global value and a value indicating patient preference for a certain desired state of health. It produces a profile of social values which together with years of life create a measure of the outcomes of medical interventions: quality-adjusted life years (QALY) [63].

EuroQol was developed simultaneously in five European countries: England, the Netherlands, Norway, Sweden and Denmark. The content was obtained from a review of the dimensions of the SIP and the Nottingham Health Profile, based on the experience of the researchers who participated in the project. The tool consist of three parts. The first is devoted to *description of health status* according to 5 dimensions (mobility, personal care, daily activities, pain/discomfort, and anxiety/depression). These dimensions are rated 1 to 3, 1 No problems, 2 Some problems, and 3 Many problems. In the second part of the test, the patient scores their state of health on a millimetre scale analogous to a 20 mm thermometer (EVA) whose extremes go from 0 (Worst State) to 100 (Best State). This EVA score can be used as a quantitative indicator of state of health. The third part is designed to obtain individual scores of preference for states designed in the descriptive part, with 14 possible states scored from 1 to 3, and in which the patient is also asked where they would place the status "death". The tool is designed to be self-administered (preferable) or through an interviewer or interviewers in patients with difficulties such as persons with visual or intellectual disabilities. It is Grade A for its psychometric criteria, for generalisability which allows studies in diverse diseases and clinical settings, and for utility of the index value in cost-effectiveness studies and especially in the allocation of clinical and care resources [29]. This questionnaire is available at http://www.euroqol.org.

4.3 Duke activity status index (DASI)

This tool was designed to analyse and assess functional capacity in cardiovascular patients based on the patient's ability to perform activities of daily living (ADLs). A version adapted to gravely hospitalised patients was also developed, based on the SUPPORT [29] study, and more recently its use was recommended as a predictor of postoperative morbidity and mortality by assessing tolerance to exercise and thus improving the planning and outcome of surgery [64]. The original questionnaire consisted of 12 items which collect information on the possibilities of performing activities of daily living (ADLs) such as personal care, mobility, household tasks and sexual functioning in the last two weeks; the reduced version does not include sexual functioning. Scores for each item range from 3 (activity performed without difficulty), 2 (activity performed with difficulty) and 1 (activity not performed for reasons of health). If a surveyed patient does not perform the activity for reasons other than health, this question is given the same score as the previous item, as it is assumed that the patient had at least the same difficulty in performing the activity. Each item has a value ranging between 1 and 2.5, such that the score ranges from 11.5 (minimum capacity) to 33 (maximum capacity). The test is designed to be self-administered (preferable because this eliminates bias) or through an interviewer or interviewers in patients with difficulties such as persons with visual or intellectual disabilities [13]. It is Grade A for its psychometric criteria of validity, reliability and sensitivity, and permits studies on cardiovascular diseases and conditions, which are among the most prevalent and primary causes of death in developed countries. Additionally, it is predictive in patients with cardiovascular disease.

4.4 General health questionnaire (GHQ)

The aim in developing this measuring tool was the detection of patients suffering from non-psychotic psychiatric disorders. It was validated for patients who requested primary care services from General Practitioners in the UK, to aid these practitioners in detecting psychiatric cases, and was later applied to epidemiological studies in the general population [29]. The questionnaire is based on the multidimensional model of the Biopsychosocial Health Model [7] and specifically for mental disorders. The author wished to distinguish between minor mental conditions and greater disorders which lead to loss of normality in connection with daily living. The tool consists of 140 items and a short 60-item form; further short forms were later developed, of which the 28-item version is the most frequently used. This last is composed of four subscales of 7 items which assess somatic symptoms of psychological origin, anxiety, difficulties in performing daily activities, and subjective perception of depression. The score for these items is 0 in responses better or equal to normal and 1 in responses worse or much worse than normal. The test is designed to be self-administered (preferable because this eliminate bias) and can be completed in under 5 minutes.

It is Grade A for its psychometric criteria of validity, reliability and sensitivity, and the 28-question version has become widely used due to the short time to administer, ease of scoring and good acceptance. Its main weakness is that it is not designed to screen for psychiatric conditions and for minor non-psychotic psychological conditions [29].

4.5 Psychological general well-being index

This survey was developed in the USA for use in community epidemiological studies as an indicator to reveal subjective feelings of well-being or psychological discomfort, i.e. for studies in the general population. The questionnaire consists of 18 items which cover 6 dimensions. The first 14 items have Likert-type answers, with six categories representing degrees of intensity or frequency which may range from 1 to 6 or from 6 to 1 depending on type of item; the remaining four items are scored on a visual analogue scale. The assessed dimensions are: anxiety, depression, positive mood, vitality, self-control and overall health. A global assessment of severe discomfort can be obtained with the lowest score, and of positive well-being with the highest. Scores can also be obtained for each dimension. A 22-item version of the tool exists which was developed by Dupay [65] for use in cardiovascular disease, and whose score ranges from 22 (patients with severe discomfort) to 132 (patients with positive well-being), which has been translated and adapted into Spanish by experts on methodology and HRQoL measurement tools [66]. It is designed to be self-administered (preferable because this eliminates bias). It is Grade A for its psychometric criteria of validity, reliability and sensitivity to change. Its main weakness is the establishing of cut-off points when differentiating between degrees of well-being: positive, negative, and severe discomfort [29].

To summarise and facilitate the analytical analysis and decision-making when choosing an instrument, these are presented in the following **Table 3**.

Instrument	Type of measure	Psychometric Indicators*	Characteristics of the more widespread versions	Utility Applicability	Recommendation
SF36	*GenericHRQoL*	*Good*	36 items/12th version 8 dimensions	*QualityofLife*	*I/SA/R*
Nottingham Health Profile	*GenericHRQoL*	*Good*	38 items 6 dimensions	Measurement of physical/ mental and social Suffering	*I/SA*
Sickness Impact Profile (SIP)	*GenericHRQoL*	*Good*	136 items/12th version 12 categories	Diseases repercussions	*SA*
EuroQol-5D	*GenericHRQoL*	*Good*	[3] parts, 8 dimensions, and Visual Scale	*Mobility, Personalcare,* *DailyActivities* *Malaise, Anxiety* Health condition	*I/SA*
Quality of Life Profile for Chronically Ill patients (PLC)	*ChronicIllnesses*	*Good*	40 items 6 dimensions	*MultidimensionalQualityofLife* Based on the concept by the WHO	*I/SA*
Duke Activity Status *Index (DASI)*	*PredictorHRQoL*	*Good*	12 items/10th version	*FunctionalCapacity* Activities of Daily Living	*SA/R*
General Health Questionnaire (GHQ-28)	*MentalHealth*	*Good*	28 items	*MentalHealth* Psychological Distress	*SA/R*
Psychological General Well-Being Index (PGWBI)	*Psychological well – being*	*Good*	22 items 6 dimensions	*Well – being∧Malaise* Psychological	*SA*

Validity, reliability /repeatability, Internal Consistency, and Sensitivity to Change.
**Interview (I), self-administered (SA) and Reference in HRQoL (R).*

Table 3.
Summary of the characteristics of the selected HRQoL instruments.

5. Conclusions

For many experts, the best indicators of the effectiveness of health services are ***indicators of Health-Related Quality of Life (HRQoL), wellbeing and citizen satisfaction***. These indicators all measure global outcomes in patients and in the population, since *quality of life and well-being* have multidimensional values and account for the perspective of the patient undergoing the clinical and/or surgical interventions, procedures and services which are recommended and prescribed by practitioners, with informed consent, such as treatment and/or functional recovery and rehabilitation.

The **generic surveys** recommended for the assessment of HRQoL as an indicator are those which grant a comprehensive perspective on patients based on the Biopsychosocial Model of Health, placing patients in the main role of the outcome.

Of these surveys, the most widely used at the international level is SF-36 due to quality criteria and because, **it is used as a reference instrument and because** and it allows more comparisons, giving greater consistency to outcomes obtained at different healthcare and social/health centres and across different countries. Alternative questionnaires exist which may be used based on patients and their health and social circumstances.

Alternative questionnaires are available such as the Nottingham Health Profile (NHP) that is better when measuring health impact in populations, or the SIP when one wants to know the perception of illness that patients refer, the main drawback being it has 136 items, thus not recommended in elderly patients. Specific questionnaires can be used based on patient characteristics. If these are chronic, the Quality of Life Profile for Chronically Ill patients (PLC) is a good option. Based on the objectives, if functional capacity is to be assessed, The *Duke* Activity Status *Index (DASI)* is valid, reliable, and sensitive. It is also predictive in patients with cardiovascular alterations, which was its first use. If you want to estimate psychological or mental well-being, the Psychological General Well-Being Index (PGWBI) is appropriate.

On the other hand, all of these questionnaires can be self-administered. Still, patient's cognitive characteristics must be taken into account, basically that they can read and understand the questions correctly so that answers are reliable.

The **goal** of using these questionnaires when assessing HRQoL is the conversion of evidence into effective results which increase patient quality of life and wellbeing, as health is a fundamental resource for life, and this requires applied or clinical research and a public health system for the improvement of quality of care, HRQoL, and wellbeing.

Author details

Jose Antonio Miron Canelo[1*], Maria-Fernanda Lorenzo Gómez[2,3], Elena Iglesias De Sena[1] and Luz Celia Fernández Martín[4,5]

1 Faculty of Medicine, Preventive Medicine and Public Health, University of Salamanca, Spain

2 Faculty of Medicine, Department of Surgery, University of Salamanca, Spain

3 Urology Department, Hospital Clínico Universitario de Salamanca, Spain

4 Faculty of Psychology, University of Salamanca, Spain

5 Psychiatry Service, Hospital Clínico Universitario de Salamanca, Spain

*Address all correspondence to: miroxx@usal.es

References

[1] Feinstein AR. Clinimetrics. New Haven: Yale University Press, 1987.

[2] Mirón Canelo JA, Alonso Sardón M. Medidas de frecuencia, asociación e impacto. Rev Medicina y Seguridad en el Trabajo 2008; 54: 93-102.

[3] Allison PJ, Locker D, Feine JS. Quality of life: a dynamic construct. Social Science and Medicine 1997; 45: 221-230.

[4] AbouZahr C, Boerma T. Los sistemas de información sanitaria, pilares de la salud pública. Boletín de la Organización Mundial de la Salud, n° 83. 2005.

[5] Galán M. Sistemas de información de Salud Pública. En: Manual de Salud electrónica para directivos de servicios y sistemas de salud. 2011: 253-271.

[6] Herdman MJ. Reflexiones sobre la medición de la calidad de vida relacionada con la Salud en España. Gac Sanit 2005; 19: 91-92.

[7] Engel G. The Need for a New Medical Model: a Challenge for Biomedicine. Science. 1977;196: 129-136.

[8] Donabedian A. Guide American Care Administration. Medical Care Appaisal-Quality and Utilization. New York, EEUU. American Public Health Association. 1969.

[9] Arahna De Macedo L, Mirón Canelo JA. Alonso Sardón M, Del Pino Montes J, Sáenz González MC. Calidad de vida relacionada con la Salud en pacientes con osteoporosis. Rev de Santé Publica de Brasil 2006; 40: 298-303.

[10] Lucas Carrasco R. Calidad de vida y demencia. Med Clin 2007;128:70-75. Doi: 10.1016/S0025-7753(07)72488-0.

[11] Mirón Canelo JA, Alonso Sardón M, Serrano López de las Hazas A, De Godos N. Sáenz González MC. Health Related Quality of Life (HRQL) in people with intellectual disability Pan Am J Public Health 2008; 24(5): 336-344.

[12] Santa Cruz Ruiz S, Mirón Canelo JA, Del Cañizo A, Santa Cruz Ruiz P. Quality of personal and social life in patients with CI. Int J Pediatric Otorhinolaryngology 2011; 75 (supl 1): 81.

[13] Alonso Sardón M, Iglesias de Sena H, Fernández Martín Luz-Celia, Mirón Canelo JA. Do health and social support and personal autonomy have an influence on the health-related quality of life of individuals with intellectual disability?. BMC Health Services Research 2019; 23;19(1):63.

[14] Flores-Fraile, Lorenzo-Gómez MF, Mirón-Canelo José-A y Otros. Impacto de la Calidad de Vida del tratamiento de Cáncer de Próstata organoconfinado. Actas Urológicas Españolas 2020; 44(9): 630-636.

[15] Nunnally JC. Psychometric Theory. New York. McGraw-Hill; 1978.

[16] Guyatt GH, ¨Should Subjects See Their Previous Responses¨. Journal Chronic Dis 1985; 38: 1003-1007.

[17] Streiner D, Norman GR. Health Measurement Scales. A practical Guide to Their Development and Use. Oxford: Osford University Press; 1995.

[18] Fletcher RH, Fletcher SW, Wagner EH. Clinical Epidemiology: The essentials. Baltimore: Williams & Williams,; 1996.

[19] Sánchez R, Gómez C. Conceptos Básicos sobre validación de escalas¨. Rev Col Psiquiatria 1998; 2: 121-130.

[20] Lantz CA, Nebenzahl E. Behavior and interpretation of the Kappa statistic: resolution of the two paradoxes. J Clin Epidemiol 1996; 49: 431-434.

[21] Krantz E, Wide U, Trimpou P, Bryman I, Landin-Wilhelmsen K. Comparison between different instruments for measuring health-related quality of life in a population sample, the WHO MONICA Project, Gothenburg, Sweden: an observational, cross-sectional study. BMJ Open. 2019 Apr 20;9(4):e024454. doi: 10.1136/bmjopen-2018-024454.

[22] Lorente S, Vives J, Viladrich C, Losilla JM. Herramientas para evaluar las propiedades de medición de los instrumentos de calidad de vida: un protocolo de meta-revisión. *BMJ Open* . 2018; 8 (7): e022829. Publicado el 23 de julio de 2018. doi: 10.1136.

[23] Alonso J, Prieto L, Antó JM. La versión española del SF 36 Health Survey (Cuestionario de Salud SF 36): un instrumento para la medida de los resultados clínicos. Med Clín (Barc) 1995; 104: 771-776.

[24] Vilagut G, Ferrer M, Rajmil L et al. El cuestionario de Salud SF 36 español: una década de experiencia y nuevos desarrollos. Gac sanit 2005; 19 (2): 135-150.

[25] Fernández García R, Sánchez Sánchez LC, López Rodríguez MM, Sánchez Granados G. Efectos de un programa de ejercicio físico y relajación en el medio acuático en pacientes con espondiloartritis: ensayo clínico aleatorizado. Med Clin 2015;145: 380-384. doi: 10.1016/j.medcli.2014.10.015

[26] Schmidt S, Vilagut G, Garin O, Cunillera O, Tresserras R, Brugulat P, Mompart A, Medina A, Ferrer M, Alonso J. Normas de referencia para el Cuestionario de Salud SF-12 versión 2 basadas en población general de Cataluña. Med Clin 2012;139: 613-25. Doi: 10.1016/j.medcli.2011.10.024

[27] Iraurgi Castillo J. Uso del índice de utilidad SF-6D en programas de mantenimiento con metadona. Med Clin 2008;131:437. doi: 10.1157/13126220.

[28] Rebollo P, Morís J, Ortega T, Valdés C, Ortega F. Estimación de un índice de utilidad mediante el uso de la versión española del Cuestionario de Salud SF-36: validez del índice SF-6D frente al EQ-5D. Med Clin 2007;128: 536-537. Doi: 10.1157/13101163

[29] Badia X, Salamamero M, Alonso J. La medida de la Salud. Guía de escalas de medición en español.· 3ª ed. Fundación Lilly. Barcelona, 2002.

[30] Gomez Pavon. Calidad de vida relacionada con la salud. La punta del iceberg del complejo abordaje de los ancianos muy mayores. Med Clin 2010; 135: 162-164. doi:10.1016/j.medcli.2009.11.025

[31] Amador-Marín B, Guerra-Martín MD. Effectiveness of non-pharmacological interventions in the quality of life of caregivers of Alzheimer. Gac Sanit. 2017 Mar-Apr;31 (2):154-160. Spanish. doi: 10.1016/j.gaceta.2016.09.006.

[32] Garzón-Maldonado FJ, Gutiérrez-Bedmar M, García-Casares N, Pérez-Errázquin F, Gallardo-Tur A, Martínez-Valle Torres MD. Health-Related quality of life in caregivers of patients with Alzheimer's disease. Neurologia. 2017 Oct;32(8):508-515.. doi: 10.1016/j.nrl.2016.02.023. Epub 2016 Apr 25.

[33] Aguirre-Camacho A, Stepanous J, Blanco-Donoso LM, Moreno-Jiménez B, Wilburn J, González-Saiz L, McKenna SP. Adaptation and Validation of the Cambridge Pulmonary Hypertension Outcome Review (CAMPHOR) for Use in Spain. Rev Esp Cardiol (Engl Ed). 2017 Jun;70(6): 467-473. doi: 10.1016/j.rec.2016.11.007

[34] Azevedo C, Pessalacia JDR, Mata LRFD, Zoboli ELCP, Pereira MDG. Interface between social support, quality of life and depression in users

eligible for palliative care. Rev Esc Enferm USP. 2017 Aug 28;51:e03245. doi: 10.1590/S1980-220X2016038003245. PMID: 28902325.

[35] García-León FJ, García-Estepa R, Romero-Tabares A, Gómez-Millán Borrachina J. Treatment of advanced laryngeal cancer and quality of life. Systematic review. Acta Otorrinolaringol Esp. 2017 Jul-Aug;68 (4):212-219. English, Spanish. doi: 10.1016/j.otorri.2016.11.005.

[36] Enríquez Reyna MC, Vargas Flores MLÁ. Factores personales que afectan la calidad de vida de mujeres con cáncer de mama del noreste de México: Personal factors that affect quality of life of women with breast cancer from the northeast of Mexico. Hisp Health Care Int. 2018 Jun;16(2):70-75. doi: 10.1177/1540415318786675.

[37] Flores-Ruvalcaba, María L. Peralta-Pedrero, Andrea De Villafranca-Dugelby, Fermín Jurado-Santa Cruz. Quality of life in adults with keloid scars. Martha A. Morales-Sánchez*, Christian N. Cir Cir 2018;86(4):321-326. doi: 10.24875/CIRU.M18000049.

[38] Muñoz-Lasa S, López de Silanes C, Atín-Arratibel MÁ, Bravo-Llatas C, Pastor-Jimeno S, Máximo-Bocanegra N. Effects of hippotherapy in multiple sclerosis: pilot study on quality of life, spasticity, gait, pelvic floor, depression and fatigue. Med Clin (Barc). 2019 Jan 18;152(2):55-58.. doi: 10.1016/j.medcli.2018.02.015.

[39] Mallolas J, Ahumada A, Ampuero J, Blanco JR, Hidalgo Á, Londoño MC, Molina E, Ruiz S. Quality of life in patients with hepatitis C. Importance of treatment. Gastroenterol Hepatol. 2019 Sep;42 Suppl 1:20-25. doi: 10.1016/S0210-5705(20)30184-9.

[40] Rørvik HD, Campos AH, Styr K, Ilum L, McKinstry GK, Brandstrup B, Olaison G. Minimal Open Hemorrhoidectomy Versus Transanal Hemorrhoidal Dearterialization: The Effect on Symptoms: An Open-Label Randomized Controlled Trial. Dis *Colon Rectum*. 2020 May;63(5): 655-667. doi: 10.1097/DCR.0000000000001588.

[41] Brazier J, Roberts J, Deveill M. The estimation of preference-based measures of health from the SF 36. Health Econ. 2002; 21:272-292.

[42] Alonso J, Antó JM, Moreno C. Spanish versión of the Nottingham Health Profile: translation and preliminary validity. Am J Public Health 1990; 80:704-708.

[43] Alonso J, Prieto L, Antó JM. The Spanish versión of the Nottingham Health Profile: a reeview of adaptation and instrument caharacteristics. Quality of Life Research 1994; 3:385-393.

[44] Prieto L, Alonso J, Viladrich MC, Antó JM. Scaling the Spanish versión of the Nottingham Health Profile: Evidence of limited value of itemweights. J of Cinical Epidemilology 1996; 49:31-38.

[45] Permanyer Miralda G, Brotons C, Cascant P, Moral I, Alonso J, Soler Soler J. Assessment of quality of life related to health 2 years after coronary surgery. Med Clin (Barc). 1997 Mar 29; 108(12):446-451.

[46] Bonfill X, Montes J, Roqué M, Nogué M, Saigi E, Seguí MA, Blanco R, Arcusa A, Arjol A, Diaz C. Evaluation prospectiva de resultados clínicos en los pacientes clínicos con cáncer de pulmón. Med Clín 2000; 114 (suppl 3): 104-111.

[47] Torrens M, San L, Garrell E, Castillo C, Martínez A, Domingo A. Use of the Nottinghal Health Profile for measurin health status of patients in methadone maintenance treatment. Addiction 1997; 92: 707-716.

[48] Bosch Romero E, Sáenz Moya N, Valls Esteve M, Viñolas Valer S. Study of quality of life of patients with fibromyalgia: impact of a health education programme. Aten Primaria. 2002 Jun 15;30(1):16-21. Spanish. doi: 10.1016/s0212-6567(02)78958-0.

[49] Lipsett PA, Swoboda SM, Campbell KA, Cornwell E 3rd, Dorman T, Pronovost PJ. Sickness Impact Profile Score versus a Modified Short-Form survey for functional outcome assessment: acceptability, reliability, and validity in critically ill patients with prolonged intensive care unit stays. J Trauma. 2000 Oct;49(4): 737-743. doi: 10.1097/00005373-200010000-00024.

[50] Prcic A, Aganovic D, Hadziosmanovic O. Sickness Impact Profile (SIP) Score, a Good Alternative Instrument for Measuring Quality of Life in Patients with Ileal Urinary Diversions. Acta Inform Med. 2013;21 (3):160-165. doi: 10.5455/aim.2013.21.160-165.

[51] Badia X, Alonso J. Validity and reproductibilityof the spanish versionof the SIP. J of Cinical Epidemiology Assessment 1996; 49:359-365.

[52] De Bruin AF, Diederiks JP, de Witte LP, Stevens FC, Philipsen H. Assessing the responsiveness of a functional status measure: the Sickness Impact Profile versus the SIP68. J Clin Epidemiol. 1997 May;50 (5):529-540. doi: 10.1016/s0895-4356 (97)00047-4.

[53] Espuña Pons M. Incontinencia de orina en la mujer. Med Clin 2003;120: 464-472.

[54] McEntee ML, Vowles KE, McCracken LM. Development of a chronic pain-specific version of the Sickness Impact Profile. Health Psychol. 2016 Mar;35(3):228-237. doi: 10.1037/hea0000257.

[55] Ferreira MC, Dias-Pereira AC, Branco-de-Almeida LS, Martins CC, Paiva SM. Impact of periodontal disease on quality of life: a systematic review. J Periodontal Res. 2017 Aug;52(4): 651-665. doi: 10.1111/jre.12436.

[56] Fernández-López JA, Hernández-Mejía R, Siegrist J. El perfil de calidad de vida para enfermos crónicos (PECVEC): un método para evaluar bienestar y funcionalismo en la práctica clínica [Quality of life profile for the chronically ill (PECVEC): a method to evaluate well-being and functioning in clinical practice]. Aten Primaria. 2001; 28(10):680-689. Spanish. doi: 10.1016/s0212-6567(01)70484-2.

[57] The EuroQol group. EuroQol: a new facility for the measurement of health related quality of life. Health Policy 1990; 16: 199-208.

[58] Badia X, Montserrat S, Herdman M, Segura A. La versión española del EuroQol: descripción y aplicaciones. Med Clin (Bar) 1999; 112(Supl 1): 79-86.

[59] Badia X, Montserrat S, Roset M, Herdman M. Feasibility, validity and test.retest realityof scaling methods for healyh states: The visual analogue scale and the time trade-off. Quality of Life Research 1999; 8(4): 303-310.

[60] Pinto JL, Lopez Lavid C, Badia X, Coma A, Benavides D. Cost effectiveness analysis of highly active antiretroviral therapy in HIV asymtomatic patients. Med Clin (Barc) 2000; 114(Supl 3):62-67.

[61] Herdman M, Badia X, Berra S. El EuroQol -5D: una alternativa sencilla para la medición de la calidad de vida relacionada con la salud en Atención Primaria. Aten Primaria 2001; 28(6): 425-430.

[62] Perona M, Mearin F, Guilera M, Mínguez M, Ortiz V, Montoro M,

Serra J, Casanova C, Rey E, Onofre Alarcón, Bujanda L, Lima A, Andreu M, Castro M, López A, Carrillo R, Sempere L, Badia X. Cuestionario específico de calidad de vida para pacientes con estreñimiento: desarrollo y validación del CVE-20. Med Clin 2008; 131: 371-377. doi: 10.1016/S0025-7753(08)72285-1.

[63] Dolan, P.; Kahneman, D. Interpretation of utility and their implications for the valuation of health. The Economic Journal. 2008;118: 215-234.

[64] Riedel B, Li MH, Lee CHA, Ismail H, Cuthbertson BH, Wijeysundera DN, Ho KM; METS Study Investigators. A simplified (modified) Duke Activity Status Index (M-DASI) to characterise functional capacity: a secondary analysis of the Measurement of Exercise Tolerance before Surgery (METS) study. Br J Anaesth. 2021 Jan; 126(1):181-190. doi: 10.1016/j.bja.2020.06.016.

[65] Dupuy HJ. Self-representations of general psycological well-being of american adults. American Public Health Association Meeting. Los Angeles CA. 1978.

[66] Badia X, Gutierrez F, Wiklund I et al. Vality and reliatbility of the spanish versión of the Generall Well-Being index. Quality Life Research 1996; 5: 101-108.

Chapter 2

Ethical Issues Which Have Prevented the U.S. from Maximizing Quality of Life Years

Sage Arbor

Abstract

The cost of healthcare interventions varies greatly with age, with a significant fraction of cost being spent in the last two years of life. Treating a child can save orders of magnitude more life-years than an octogenarian treated for the same disease, such as cancer. While Quality-Adjusted Life Years (QALYs) can be used to plan a roadmap for how resources should be expended to maximize quality of life the execution of those plans often fail due to societal norms which trump the carefully measured QALYs, resulting in lowered average number and/or quality of years lived. The ethical issues concerning age, sex, lifestyle (smoking, drinking, obesity), cost transparency, and extreme examples (war, population explosion vs. collapse) will be discussed.

Keywords: Quality Adjusted Life Years (QALY), generation, elder care, disability-adjusted life year (DALY), fair innings, rule of rescue, standard gamble, cost transparency, organ donation, smoking, alcoholism, diabetes

1. Introduction

Quality Adjusted Life Years (QALYs) provide a quantified mechanism to alot limited healthcare resources to maximize desired years and quality of life. Both the numbers of years we live and the quality of health has increased more in the last 150 years than in any prior time in human history. It is interesting that QALYs were invented at the same time the variables that go into defining QALYs are changing so rapidly. The U.S. National Council on Disability (NCD) has found sufficient evidence that QALYs are discriminatory by design, and suggested Congress should pass legislation prohibiting the use of QALYs by Medicaid and Medicare [1]. What constitutes a disability and how much should it decrease QALYs? There have been deaf families that argue deafness is not a disability, it heightens other senses, and have chosen not to have cochlear implants. What QALY hit do paraplegics receive compared to quadriplegics? The very nature of QALYs cause users to assign some agreed upon weights to life abilities.

The average human lifespan has increased 80% over the last 120 years, with a clear increase in longevity starting at the end of the 19th century (around 1890). Those living in the United Kingdom, increased average lifespan from 45.2 to 81 years from 1890 to 2015. The United States had a similar increase, doing slightly less well recently with an average lifespan of 79 in 2015. The global average lifespan started from a lower level with its significant increase delayed a decade (1900) but has paralleled the gains each year achieving even more impressive results, starting at 32 years in 1900 and rising to 71.7 years in 2015 [2] (**Figure 1**). Starting in the 20th Century infant mortality plummeted from 10% to under 1% currently, which significantly contributed to the average lifespan. However, if you look at mortality rates at later ages it is apparent that lifespan has increased after keeping infants alive [3]. There is significant scientific data now that, across the animal kingdom, caloric restriction extends life [4–9] which provided hope we could continue the trend increasing human longevity. In mice a 60% reduction in calories has been shown to increase lifespan by about a third, however in humans and primates it appears we may only be able to extend our lives 1–5 years [10, 11] though research is ongoing [12].

It has been estimated that while clinical care accounts for 15% of the quality of one's health, clinical care data only represents 0.1% of the data (0.4 terabytes) applicable to health outcomes over their lifetime (1,106 terabytes) [13]. Most of the data that affects one's health (1,100 terabytes) concerns one's social determinants of health and health behaviors which account for 40% and 20% of one's quality of health respectively. The last 25% of one's health is determined by "Nonmodifiable factors" such as genetics, but this data (6 terabytes) is still very actionable in that different actions (e.g. pharmaceuticals, diet, lifestyle interventions) can be taken based on one's genetics. While it is likely most easy to modify healthcare's actions in clinical care, because it only represents 15% of our health outcomes, in order to maximize QALYs we must invest in analyzing and modifying the other data realms that affect our lifetime biomedical health (social determinants of health, health behaviors, and nonmodifiable factors).

Medical spending has increased by an order of magnitude in the last 200 year as a proportion of GDP. The share of GDP used on healthcare in 1800, 1850, 1900, 1950, 200o was 2%, 2.1%, 2.5%, 4.5%, 13.5% respectively (**Figure 1**) [14]. There is a clear and historically long trend of healthcare accounting for larger percentages of GDP in the developing world. Despite concern that this increased expenditure is just going to fatten the profits of big pharma, the reality is more nuanced with significantly more people and services being funded. Concomitantly and unsurprisingly, in the U.S. rapid growth is projected in both health and STEM occupations

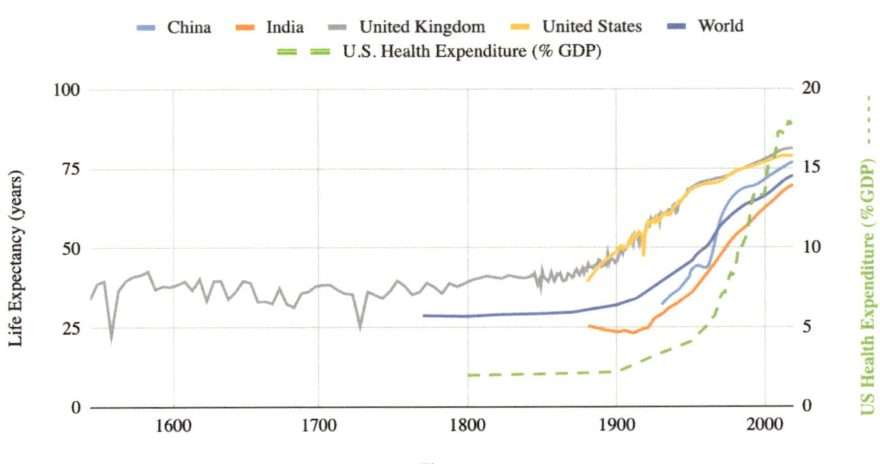

Figure 1.
Life Expectancy and Expenditure on Healthcare increase over time. Source: Our World in Data. https://ourworldindata.org/life-expectancy.

while office support, food service, and manufacturing production jobs will decline [1]. In order to maintain or lower the cost of healthcare, country's must either lower costs per treatment (increased efficiency) or reduce treatment provided (decreased expenditure). While everyone would like the former solution of getting the same treatment for cheaper, the continual rise in healthcare expenditures despite plateauing lifespan suggests cuts will be needed. There are large economic differences in healthcare expenditures between countries which do not translate to better care. Common examples are the United States spending 10-fold more per citizen than Cuba despite similar life expectancies. The counties of the E.U. also spend less than the United States while having the same or better life spans. The successes and failures of using QALYs to reduce healthcare costs will be discussed. Most of the QALY issues discussed apply globally. However, this chapter will focus on data and issues in the United States, which is unusual among industrialized countries because it does not have a single payer system, and therefore has uniquely heightened QALY misallocations.

1.1 QALYs vs. DALYs

In 1976 Zeckhauser and Shepard first used the term Quality-Adjusted Life Years (QALYs) to describe measurements of health outcomes which were defined by both duration and quality of life measurements [15]. Pliskin detailed the three assumptions QALYs required to act as valid metrics to assign health resources [16], namely:

1. Independence between health status and life years

2. A constant proportional trade-off

3. Risk neutrality of life years

While these foundational assumptions of QALYs have been questioned [17], they have been globally accepted and used by most countries for making economic decisions [18–21].

Two decades after the description of a QALY, the Disability-Adjusted Life Years (DALYs) were developed in the 1990s measuring both duration as well as quality. DALYs by definition measure disease burden but are also often used like QALYs to maximize cost-effectiveness. QALYs have a health-related quality of life weighting (Q) that ranges from 0 to 1, with 1 representing a year of perfect health and 0 representing death. A Q measure of 0.5 has been expressed as bed ridden, and it should be noted that a state considered "worse" than death can have a negative Q rating. The quality of life each year can be added up to calculate one's quality-adjusted life expectancy (QALE). On the other hand DALYs are measured from 0 to 1 where 0 represents no disability. Therefore in QALYs the higher the weighting the better, but in DALYs the lower the weighting the better. Usually expert valuations are assigned to a universal set of weightings for DALYs, whereas QALYs use preference-based health-related measures gathered from groups of patients or the general population [22]. DALYs have an age-weighting function, and can therefore preferentially favor spending money on the young versus the old compared to QALYs.

- QALYs lived in one year = 1*Q (where $Q \leq 1$)

$$QALEt = \sum_{t}^{t+RLE} Qt$$

Q_t = Health related quality of life weighting at year t.
QALE = quality-adjusted life expectancy at a given age.
RLE = Residual Life Expectancy at given age.
t = individual years within residual life expectancy range.

2. Equity - is each year of perfect life equal?

As QALYS are used to determine the allotment of financial resources, the age of the citizens receiving these resources can be a significant issue. The most common causes of death in the U.S. (stroke, cancer, Chronic Lower Respiratory Diseases (CLRD), Alzheimers, heart disease, and diabetes) debilitate patients for a broad duration, ranging from immediate death to 20 years (**Table 1**, **Figure 2**). Death can occur suddenly with almost no recourse for intervention or financial expenditure by society aimed to improve life, such as in an unforeseen and lethal suicide or stroke. However, disease care is becoming more often a case of extended managed care, such as with diabetes.

2.1 Old vs. Young

2.1.1 Fair innings

The philosophical framework termed "fair innings" posits that each human has an equal right to experience each phase (age) of life. Therefore if the same intervention could extend for one year the life of a 60-year-old or a 26-year-old, then the younger patient should preferentially get the intervention so they have their "fair-inning" at

Disease	Total Deaths (million, U.S. 2017)	Deaths/100,000 (U.S. 2017)	Deaths/100,000 (U.S. 2007)	Change 2007–2017 (% change)	Average duration of disease
Heart disease	647	165	190.9	−13.6	7.3 yrs
Cancer	599	152.5	178.4	−14.5	2 yrs
Chronic lower respiratory diseases (CLRD)	160	40.9	40.8	0	4 yrs
Stroke	146	37.6	43.5	−13.6	1 yr
Alzheimer disease	121	31	22.7	36.6	6 yrs
Diabetes	84	21.5	22.5	−4.4	30 yrs
Influenza and pneumonia	56	14	15.7	−10.8	1.5 weeks
Kidney disease	51	13	15.7	−17.2	7 yrs
Suicide	47	14	11.3	23.9	1 day

Data was retrieved from the National Vital Statistics Reports Final Death Reports. The color coding represents better values in green (low deaths, low disease duration, and decreased deaths over time) adn worse values in red.
https://pubmed.ncbi.nlm.nih.gov/25075874/
https://pubmed.ncbi.nlm.nih.gov/32501199/

Table 1.
Duration of Disease vs. Population Effect.

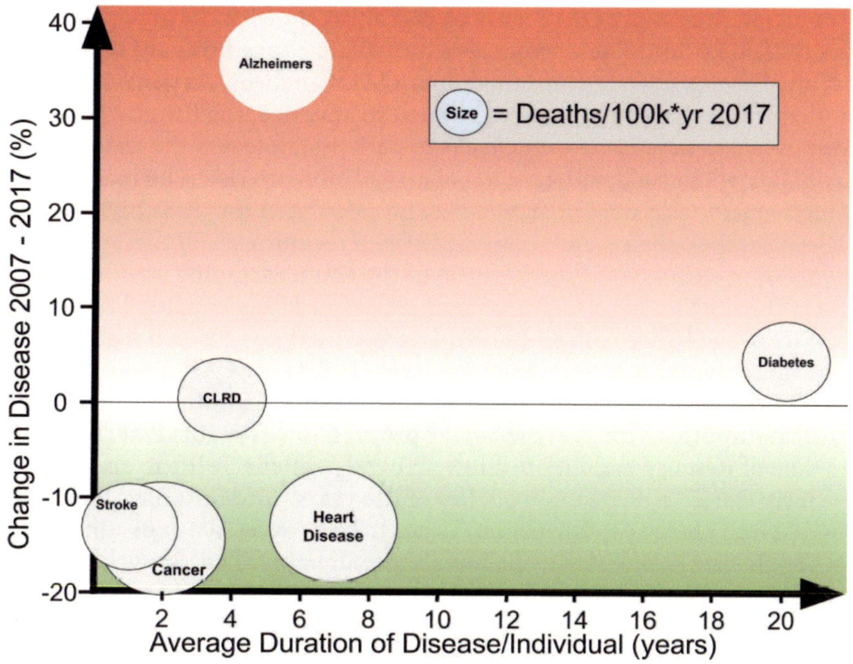

Figure 2.
Length of Public Health Issues vs. Population Effect.

living the age of 27. Human lifespan has roughly doubled in the last century, from roughly 40 to 80 years of life in the developed world. Does a child that is born into the world that now lives 10% longer than their parents have the scaled protection to get to the world's future average lifespan (10% older than their parents), or do fair innings apply as a static set of years based on the oldest generations having care rationed? If nations had been rationing care based on the "fair innings" philosophy they would have possibly undervalued young years of life if they were not taking into account the projected increase in lifespan for younger generations. Recently the lifespan in the United States decreased for the first time in decades due to a combination of macro health issues (obesity, opiod overdose, and suicide epidemics). While the current U.S. healthcare system does not ration care based on fair innings principles, if it had done so and taken into account the longstanding historical increases in lifespan younger generations would have received more resources than deemed fair in hindsight since their projected lifespan has dropped from historical trends. One of the most important aspects for implementing allotment of healthcare resources based on QALYs is for the electorate to have supreme confidence in its fairness. The use of fair innings is very transparent in taking from one group (older) to give to another group (younger), and any projection based on moving average lifespans could increase the publics distrust in QALY use for policy decisions.

2.1.2 Rule of Rescue

In 1986 Albert Jonsen coined the term "Rule of Rescue" which described the medical community's unwillingness to allow patients to die, even when a high cost to save them made the QALY calculation suggest the resources would be better used elsewhere [23]. Jonsen described examples of sitting on various committees to decide the value of interventions (artificial heart, cardiac transplantation, amniocentesis, liver transplant, autologous bone marrow transplantation), and a recurring theme emerged in which the debate would go down a consistent path detailing the high cost per QALY only to end abruptly with the group deciding the lives must be saved. These expensive transplant procedures are still covered in the United States despite continued poor QALY analysis. As genetic knowledge and biomedical technologies have continued to advance, the list of expensive procedures that deliver increased QALYs to patients, however the absolute cost and % of GDP spent on healthcare has also continued to rise. The incremental cost effectiveness ratio per QALY needs to be calculated for these high ticket items. For example, the recent chimeric antigen receptor T cell therapy (CAR-T therapy) [24] appears cost effective 95% of the time, assuming a willingness to pay $100,000 USD for each QALY gained, despite costing roughly half a million dollars USD in the United States (depending on the type of B-cell malignancy) [25]. The incremental cost-effectiveness ratio (ICER) for CAR-T was found to be somewhere between roughly $64,000/QALY and $175,000 depending on the study and assumptions for average 5-year progression-free survival (PFS) [25–27].

The Rule of Rescues inability to allow an overly expensive life to end has resoundingly caused a decrease in quality of life years. Attempts have been made over the last half century in the United States to limit excessive expenditures for care during the last two years of life, but almost all have failed. Some have argued the rule of rescue is defensible even from a utilitarian point of view in that the citizenry will have increased "well-being" because they desire living in a community that values life, and while that trend is likely true it cannot defend the rule of rescue without bounds [28]. Most see the rule of rescue as contradicting the utilitarian nature of QALY optimization for healthcare expenditures.

The Affordable Care Act (ACA, also known as Obamacare) was the greatest leap towards universal coverage in the United States in the last 50 years (since Medicaid was signed into law in 1965), but is not close to the single payer systems that Europe has long implemented. The ACA initially proposed paying physicians if they provided voluntary counseling to Medicare patients about end-of-life care options, advance directives, or living wills. During the 2009 presidential debate Sarah Palin famously termed these clauses "death panels" describing a future where doctors decided whose parents would die. These aspects of the bill were removed before final passage as result of public pressure.

2.1.3 Standard gamble

The standard gamble is a more patient specific measure of if a medical intervention should be done. **Figure 3** shows a simple standard gamble in which a health intervention could result in either a better or worse outcomes than no intervention (e.g. an organ transplant). The probability p of the best outcome (healthy), is changed until the patient has no preference over whether to get the medical intervention or not, at which point their personalized standard gamble has been calculated [22]. There are other standard gamble scenarios/diagrams when, for example, no outcome results in death, or any intervention outcome is higher than lack of intervention.

2.2 Women vs. Men

2.2.1 Pregnancy

Should a pregnant woman in need of care have QALYs counted for herself and her baby, just herself, just her baby, and how does the age of the fetus change that calculus? If one adheres to the "fair innings" paradigm (see above), then the early years of a newborn are more valuable than the mothers later years. It seems clear that if a female near term needed resources her QALY measurement should, at a minimum, be the

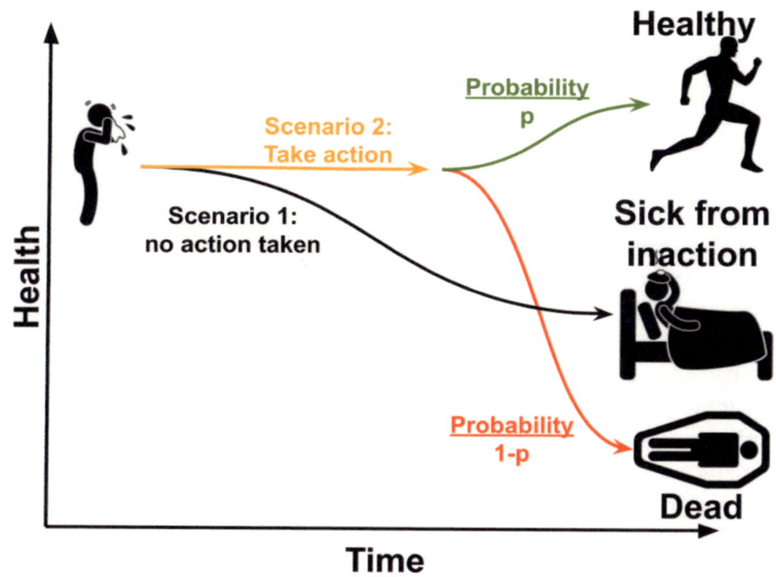

Figure 3.
Standard Gamble.

greater childs QALYs if fair innings were being taken into account. QALYs are often not scaled by age (no fair innings implementation) and the pregnant female would have resources assigned worth double a single person (with equal weight for her and her child). In reality there are often not even the attempted use of QALYs in such situations in the United States, because lethal pregnancy issues are handled like other Emergency Department critical patients following the rule of rescue (see above) in that any resources are used to save the lives at that moment. Costs of infertility treatment share many of these same QALY accounting issues, and have other societal/ethical issues in addition. For example, early this century the UK 's National Institute for Clinical Excellence (NICE) covered infertility costs but explicitly excluded "social infertility" which includes a woman being single or homosexual. Under that paradigm a woman 40 years of age that has fertility issues could qualify for in vitro fertilization (IVF) over a woman half her age that happens to be single and/or a lesbian [29]. Similarly to how the rule of rescue trumps all other QALY calculations, societal norms can have a trumping effect of completely removing groups from medical coverage. A common delimiter for excluding a group from medical coverage is if there is a nonmedical lifestyle action/intervention to effect the same increase in QALYs, such as finding a male spouse in the above example. To the authors' knowledge no country has seriously addressed this issue in any way other than looking at them on a case by case basis by a panel (e.g. by health experts, philosophers, politicians).

2.2.2 Sex lifespan differences

Women live longer than men across the globe (~8% or 6 years). Roughly $100,000 USD more is spent on women's health than men during their life ($375,000 $275,000). Since healthcare later in life is more expensive this translates to women costing society more as they live longer during an expensive healthcare phase. Roughly half (45%) of women's increased healthcare costs come just from this longer lifespan. However individual situations could have calculations suggesting women get more than parity in resources. For example, if 50-year-old male and a 51-year-old female needed the same resource (such as an organ transplant) the longer female lifespan could suggest even a slightly older woman should take precedence over her junior male counterpart.

3. Organ Donor Waitlist

The transplant of organs could theoretically have extremely positive QALY returns per dollar spent, depending on the age. There are a plethora of ethical issues that arise from organ donations however, such as how important is the patient's age, their relation to the organ donor, the duration of organ viability after transplantation, or the degree to which their personal actions resulted in their need for an organ transplant.

If a young child in need of an organ could live a full life time with one transplant the QALY calculations would likely result in societies funding these transplants without any second guessing. Indeed curably treating young patients with a lethal disease is the best scenario to maximize QALYs gained, if comparing similarly priced interventions. However, organ transplants often do not alleviate a patient's disease for a normal lifespan. For example, cystic fibrosis (CF) patients most often die from lung failure due to thick mucus and biofilm accumulation leading to necrosis of the tissue. Lung transplants are done for CF patients but transplants usually only perform sufficiently for 5 years. CF patients can now live over 40 years, double the 20 year lifespan they had half a century ago. Therefore, contrary to other QALY based interventions, transplants are not recommended for the younger CF patients.

While most donated organs come from donors after they have died, there are also living organ donations. Directed living organ donation, the most common type as opposed to non-directed organ donation, allows the donor to choose the recipient (often a family member) [30]. Even the most rigorous ordering of donor recipients using rankings to maximize QALYs can suddenly be shortcut by directed living organ donors. This is an example where there is a limited supply (of organs) and the calculations to maximize QALYs changes because a family member is willing to increase that limited supply but only if used in the manner they want. Therefore there are times when a healthcare system can increase QALYs at the sacrifice of absolute ethical parity of all patients based on their need.

Smokers receiving lung transplants is another case example highlighting societies' concern about funding healthcare solutions for ailments which has been self-inflicted. More than a third of lung transplants in the U.S. are for former smokers (40%), but they often only qualify once they have proven they have quit smoking. This achieves two outcomes. Most quantifiably it increases QALYs in that a lung transplant given to someone who will never smoke again, will on average produce more QALYs than if the lung transplant were given to someone that immediately starts smoking multiple packs a day after surgery. It also addresses the moral issue, allowing the donor and society to feel like the gift of the organ is being valued by the recipient. However one study showed after smokers receive lung transplants 11% admitted they resumed smoking, with another 6% showing high levels of urinary cotinine (a metabolite of nicotine). These values are similar to heart and renal transplant recipients, who reported smoking after transplantation at a frequency of 21% and 25% respectively [31].

4. Self-inflicted medical issues

4.1 Smokers

There are many health issues for which the individual is primarily responsible. Smoking and alcoholism may be the best examples. A recent study showed that cessation of smoking alone could save up to 12 years of life [32]. Should the population that lives a healthier lifestyle pay for the less healthy lifestyle chosen by other individuals? Even cases that seem extremely clear, such as smoking, are often more complicated. For example, those living in Beijing, China have the exposure equivalent to smoking 25 cigarettes per day, just from breathing in the high particulate air [33, 34]. It seems unfair to not cover the respiratory issues of a child born in Bejing, just because those same respiratory issues are self-induced by a heavy smoker in the countryside.

4.2 Alcoholism

For a decade scientific papers appeared to show low levels of alcohol could be beneficial, with people pointing to the resveratrol in wine as an epigenetic antiaging molecule, or the blue zones of the world that consumed red wine such as Italy. In reality their high fish, high vegetable, and low calorie diet are greater life prolonging life styles. It also turns out in many of these studies the alcohol "abstainer" groups had prior alcoholics included in them, who had previously changed their lifestyle to never consume alcohol. While the abstainer group had slightly poorer health than the one drink a day group, it is likely that could be due to prior damage the alcoholics had done to their body before becoming abstainers. Such scientific errors will cause resources to be misallocated if QALYs are used coarsely to allocate every dime of resource. Should alcoholics be required to quit drinking before receiving a liver transplant? Is one drink a day ok for them. One drink a day should be physically ok for the transplanted liver, but could cause the patient to slip and start drinking heavily again. Heavy alcohol consumption clearly causes cirrhosis of the liver, however contrary to the lay public's view this is the second leading cause of cirrhosis (while hepatitis C is the leading cause) [35]. Not publicly funding healthcare for self-induced ailments clearly could save significant percentages of healthcare expenditures. However, it could lead to patients lying about their health habits and is difficult to implement fairly given the multimodal hazards for multiple diseases.

4.3 Diabetes

Diabetes and Alzheimer disease are two of the most serious medical conditions the developed world must grapple with. Both diseases are increasing rapidly in the population, while patients are able to live with the conditions for over a decade. Alzheimer's will not be discussed as there are excellent reviews of the issues [36–38], but in short it poses a problem in that there is no treatment on the horizon. Diabetes (type II) on the other hand is extremely targetable, with reduced caloric consumption and exercise literally at the patients finger tips. However, both of these solutions have some socioeconomic interacting factors. Wealthier people can afford the time for leisure exercise, and can buy more expensive but healthier food that is less calorically dense (e.g. fresh vegetables). Some of these caveats are not as pernicious as they sound. While some fresh vegetables can be expensive and perishable, frozen vegetables, potatoes, and legumes are all healthy and cheap with a long shelf life. In addition, while difficult, anyone can choose to "just eat less" which actually has a negative cost. The true social cost to reduced calorie intervention is in building and supporting structures to increase the success rate obese individuals have in transitioning from an unhealthy to healthy lifestyle.

Are genetic predispositions a disability? Generally any inherited disorder is more likely to have healthcare solutions funded for it than self-imposed maladies. Historically these inherited disabilities have been very binary, e.g. an extreme life threatening autosomal recessively inherited disease in which a child had the poor misfortune, 25% chance, of getting both deleterious alleles from their mom and dad. However we are now getting genetic knowledge that a person is only predisposed to ailments, which often have environmental causes as well. For example obese grandparents can pass on epigenetic modifications to their grandchildren that makes them 4-fold more likely to be diabetic. Is that a self-induced ailment? The grandparents might have caused their metabolic disorder by overeating, but the grandchildren clearly started birth with a biological handicap.

Hemodialysis, the most common form of dialysis, performs the kidneys function by taking a patient's blood through a filter outside of their body (cleaning it), and then returning it to their body. Dialysis is a one of the most common, expensive, and recurring treatments in developed countries, with diabetics greatly predisposed to need treatment [39]. Diabetics, by definition, cannot control their blood glucose levels and their kidneys are therefore working overtime to continually secrete excess sugar from the blood, often ending in organ failure. Early type II diabetics (<5 years of disease) do not cost society a lot in healthcare, with depression being the costliest comorbidity (64–82% increase). However, the later nonfatal complications have much larger increases in healthcare costs: end-stage renal disease with dialysis (201–599%), hemorrhagic/ischemic stroke (37–376%), and amputation of upper/lower-extremities (13–279%). Fatal complications had even larger cost increases with cardiovascular death being the most expensive (1,784–2,001%), but "other-cause deaths" being costly as well (1,285–1,584%) [40]. The rule of rescue makes these later expensive interventions covered, while spending that money on prevention earlier would save more QALYs/$.

5. Extreme examples affecting QALYs

When assigning QALYs gained by a medical intervention both the duration of extra time lived and the quality of that time need to be measured, with the former being a much easier/reproducible value to calculate. There are many extreme health scenarios (e.g. wars, population changes, climate change, paradigm shifts creating seemingly unlimited resources) that are useful examples to walk through when considering how QALYs should be measured and used to alot resources.

5.1 War

Warfare represents an extreme environment in which both the broad and mortal health need can bring clarity to how we perform our healthcare resource allocation decisions. During war the local healthcare capability can change quickly as resources are stressed both geographically and temporally. Medical triage during war is needed to use the limited medical personal and resources for those most likely to benefit from that care. In extreme examples this can include neglecting dying patients who could be saved during less strenuous times.

Medics are viewed as more important because they can in the immediate future save more lives. The future potential of one to increase QALYs of others is a thorny topic. How far in the future can you predict this and how certain do you need to be? The argument has been made that richer people that own companies could have more highly weighted QALYs because they employ others, raise the Gross Domestic Product (GDP), which causes a greater tax base to contribute more taxes towards the healthcare infrastructure therefore increasing the resources to improve QALYs. Such an argument clarifies a known tradeoff when measuring and using QALYs: there are times when a known method to increase QALYs is openly not desired or acted on because of the consensus that it would not be fair. Therefore, while QALYs are usually presented in a completely utilitarian view, their implementation openly breaks this at will when there is a consensus that the increased utility would come at the cost of equality for the program's participants. This favoring of fairness over utility may be because the equality or lack thereof is apparent immediately at each decision point, whereas the utility gain is often deferred temporally (sometimes as long as decades into the future).

5.2 Population explosion vs. collapse

The value assigned to a new human life can change during an individual's life or as a society evolves. Early in life people may not be ready to care for a child and choose to terminate pregnancies, saving their resources for the average 1–3 children they want to have later in their life. As nations become more wealthy their population chooses to have less children, investing more resources in the quality of each life. In the last two centuries human population has grown exponentially. If the total sum of QALYs were measured over that time, the last 200 years, they would clearly also follow a similar, and likely steeper, exponential increase. Not only has lifespan increased but quality of life has increased. While people are unaware of how much life has improved [41], poverty and related health issues have decreased outside the first world nations during the last 50 years [42].

5.2.1 Climate catastrophe

With the rising global population and use of fossil fuels, there has been a causal rise in the global warming gas carbon dioxide (CO_2). Earth CO_2 atmospheric levels are now at 418 parts per million (ppm), a third higher than they were after world war II. Deleterious climate effects have already occurred [43] (e.g. acidification of the ocean, bleaching of coral reefs, sea level rise submerging island nations, increased hurricane activity, droughts, crop loss, famine). In 2006 Patz and Olson estimated that climate change had already caused 5,000,000 DALYs in a 30 year timeframe, which was mostly burdened by the developing countries [44]. Scientists are even more concerned about future tipping points which the earth would be unlikely to recover from for many decades. Recently Schneider et al. showed a level of 1,200 ppm CO_2 could cause the disappearance of climate cooling clouds covering the ocean and result in 8°C (14F) rise in global temperature [45]. Such a dramatic change would melt all of Greenland and much (if not all) of Antarctica's glaciers, raising sea level and flooding all coastal cities globally, in which roughly 20% of the world's population lives.

When millions, or billions, of humans are affected by such a foreseeable super event the weightings of actionable paths forward often have large ranges of uncertainty. What is the likelihood of such an event happening and of suggested interventions preventing the negative effects? What will be the health consequences of such a large portion of the earth having to relocate. The situation becomes more dire the faster the migration of people has to happen. While sea level rise is universally understandable and viewable, a faster and perhaps more pernicious effect will likely be rising air temperature. While humans are amazingly adaptable to different temperature zones we do have an upper temperature limit, the wet-bulb temperature (TW) of 35°C (95°F). Above this temperature humans cannot shed heat, and if a region attained this temperature for extended periods it would be impossible for humans to live there without air conditioning. In a business-as-usual emission model, Representative Concentration Pathway (RCP) 8.5, parts of the Middle East and South Asia could regularly exceed this 35°C threshold in the near future [46–48]. Deaths have not historically been cataloged at or above this 35°C limit because lethal issues can occur before that temperature limit is reached. In 2020 Raymond et al. reviewed weather stations globally and found many TW around 31°C and two stations above the human limit of 35°C [49]. Most of these temperatures occurred for short periods, 1–2 hours, but a fearsome spike in TW was found to occur in some coastal locations where an afternoon breeze could bring in humidity from the water spiking the wet bulb temperature. Dubai is already planning a city that will be enclosed in a dome, called "Mall of the World" and cover 48 million square feet while taking 10 years to complete. This domed city would protect the citizenry from inhospitable heat, while acting in a second fashion as a place to study a closed ecosystem with an eye towards building cities on the moon or mars.

5.2.2 Small populations

The value societies assign to growing their population can vary for a myriad of reasons, such as predominant religious doctrine. There has been recent excitement about human travel to the moon and mars, with permanent settlement on the latter. If there were a mars base with less than 10,000 people the QALY analysis to save a newborn compared to a 80 year old would likely be different than the same question on earth. In this thought experiment the fair innings would likely trump the rule of rescue on Mars when assigning health resources to young vs. old.

5.2.3 Unlimited resources

In the next 50–100 years humanity may have nearly unlimited resources: energy (e.g. solar panels, fusion) and robotics/machines to perform the necessary tasks for humans to thrive (e.g. farming food, building shelter, developing and raising children). Under such a paradigm the younger generation is not an imposition on older generations so there would not be as much of a downside to increasing birth rates. Humanity has historically seemed insatiable in its use of resources so such a paradigm may never arise, but if it did for even a few generations (somewhat like fossil fuels did for energy use at times) then QALYs would have to be fought over less as the world would be less of a zero sum game.

These extreme examples point out that QALYs between groups are useful to view how resources are assigned in different situations, highlighting societal norms that can override QALY analysis. It is fairly easy to determine the Life Years (LY) saved when measuring a QALY, harder to measure the Quality (Q), and perhaps hardest to incorporate the QALY to limit resource use in one area compared to another when confronted by societal norms that push against this.

6. Cost transparency

6.1 Insurance deductions

A common modern occurrence in the United States is for an insured patient to receive a medical bill in which over 90% of the cost has been deducted through agreements between the insurance company and the medical supplier. The remaining bill is paid by the insurance company and the patients copay, or by the patient if they haven't met their deductible limit. With people's healthcare plan changing annually in the U.S. for multiple reasons (e.g. loss of job, changing job, moving to a different state, employer change in plan options, change in medical conditioning warranting upgrading or downgrading coverage), patients realistically rarely know the cost of medically covered procedures prior to obtaining care.

DOI: http://dx.doi.org/10.5772/intechopen.97561

6.2 Care across health systems

In the United States the lack of universal healthcare or a single payer system makes it harder to collect data on where and what healthcare dollars are being spent on. Large hospital systems are much better at measuring costs and expenditures within their network, than cities are at measuring the same across multiple networks. As an example between 2002 and 2016 patients with Heart Failure (HF) had a decrease in mortality (6.8% to 4.9%) and length of stay in a hospital (8.6 to 6.5 days) respectively. However they had an increase in cost per stay ($14,301 to $17,925) due to more extensive complications and procedures during the stay. At the same time their post-hospital expenses went up from 2002 to 2016 including discharge to long-term care (20.8% to 25.6%) [50]. Hospitals can save money by getting patients out the door quickly, but the society and patients are worse off if they leave the hospital only to encounter greater expenses and long-term discharge times.

6.3 Balanced budgets

The United States has held a privileged position in the world (militarily, financially, and societally) since the end of the second world war. Financially the U.S. has been able to borrow money both domestically and through foreign funds as the US dollar has been held as the global reserve currency. At times, such as during the Clinton presidency (1993–2001) there was economic prosperity and balanced budgets, at which time you see a leveling off of healthcare expenditure by %GDP (**Figure 1**). However, the vast majority of years the U.S. Congress has not been able to pass a balanced budget. This has allowed the U.S. to spend more on healthcare then there is money for, putting this debt on future generations. Perhaps the electorate would demand more of their elected officials if when economic successes were conveyed in the media they were scaled by how much debt was taken on to achieve them. For example, if healthcare coverage was increased by spending $X more for services, but that was during a year where the deficit (or borrowed money) was 20% higher than revenues, then the reported success should only be in funding a 80% * $X increase in healthcare support. The U.S. Revenue has been around 17% of GDP for the past 30 years, while spending has averaged about 20%. While congress has historically worried about deficits in the capital-B range (Billions) of US dollars, during the covid-19 pandemic both the Trump and succeeding Biden administration had relief packages in the capital-T (Trillion) dollar range. The fact that states generally keep balanced budgets, since they don't have the legal means to print money like the fed, has kept future medical debt from being much worse.

6.4 Surgical decisions

Hospital administration, physicians, and patients can choose a very expensive procedure/surgery based on a perceived outcome which does not match the scientific outcome data. This misalignment can occur when a decision needs to be made quickly, the intervention has a positive short term outcome compared to longer term issue (such as reducing immediate pain), or for financial reasons if the hospital stands to benefit from a procedure covered by insurance. An example is the increase in the United States of C-section deliveries, compared to vaginal births, which rose from ~20% in the late 1990s to over 30% 15 years later [51]. In 2010 cesarean deliveries were 40% more expensive than vaginal deliveries, $9,905 versus $7,089 respectively [52]. Cesarean deliveries can reduce the incidence of pelvic floor disorders

(PFD), namely stress urinary incontinence (SUI) and pelvic organ prolapse (POP), but the future savings do not offset the larger increase in delivery costs. The rate of SUI and POP after a vaginal birth are 13% and 14% respectively, but drop to 7% and 5% respectively after a cesarean birth. While the cost of surgeries for POP and SUI are expensive ($6,878 and $10,600 respectively) the relatively rare occurrence causes the average savings ($344 and $742 respectively) to be dwarfed by the higher delivery cost ($2,816) [52].

7. Conclusions

Human lifespan has doubled over the last 150 years, with the quality of those extra years also rising. However, the % of GDP spent on healthcare has more than doubled at a rate that is unsustainable to continue for the next 150 years. The concept of using QALYs to maximize quality with limited resources has gained acceptance in countries throughout the world. The country's (e.g. in the E.U) with single payer systems are better situated to measure QALYs and use them to maximize quality of care compared to the United States. Societal norms, such as Rule of Rescue, prevent the maximum use of QALYs. The lack of transparency to prices and the ease with which the U.S. can borrow money has both made the use of QALYs difficult. As the costs, outcomes, and options of clinical interventions are made more clear and accessible to society writ large, the cost of healthcare can be lowered and average quality increased at a national level.

Conflict of interest

The authors declare no conflict of interest.

Appendices and nomenclature

ACA	Affordable Care Act (also known as Obamacare)
CAR-T	Chimeric Antigen Receptor T-cell therapy
CLRD	Chronic Lower Respiratory Disease
DALY	Disability Adjusted Life Year
IVF	In Vitro Fertilization
NCD	National Council on Disability
NICE	UK's National Institute for Clinical Excellence
GDP	Gross Domestic Product
HF	Heart Failure
PFD	Pelvic Floor Disorder
POP	Pelvic Organ Prolapse
ppm	Parts Per Million
QALE	Quality Adjusted Life Expectancy
QALY	Quality Adjusted Life Year
RCP	Representative Concentration Pathway
SUI	Stress Urinary Incontinence
USD	United States Dollar

DOI: http://dx.doi.org/10.5772/intechopen.97561

Author details

Sage Arbor
Marian University College of Medicine, Indianapolis, IN, USA

*Address all correspondence to: sagearbor@gmail.com

References

[1] Romano N, Ogunyipe B, Altom B, Belt R, Brett J, Gade D, et al. Quality-Adjusted Life Years and the Devaluation of Life with a Disability [Internet]. National Council on Disability (NCD); 2019 Nov [cited 2020 Nov 16]. (Bioethics and Disability Series.). Available from: http://www.bioethics.net/2019/11/quality-adjusted-life-years-and-the-devaluation-of-life-with-a-disability-2/

[2] Roser M, Ortiz-Ospina E, Ritchie H. Life Expectancy. Our World in Data [Internet]. 2013 May 23 [cited 2020 Nov 16]; Available from: https://ourworldindata.org/life-expectancy

[3] Bongaarts J, Feeney G. How Long Do We Live? Population and Development Review. 2002;28(1):13-29.

[4] López-Lluch G, Navas P. Calorie restriction as an intervention in ageing. J Physiol. 2016 Apr 15;594(8):2043-2060.

[5] Mercken EM, Crosby SD, Lamming DW, JeBailey L, Krzysik-Walker S, Villareal D, et al. Calorie restriction in humans inhibits the PI3K/AKT pathway and induces a younger transcription profile. Aging Cell. 2013 Aug;12(4):645-651.

[6] Redman LM, Smith SR, Burton JH, Martin CK, Il'yasova D, Ravussin E. Metabolic Slowing and Reduced Oxidative Damage with Sustained Caloric Restriction Support the Rate of Living and Oxidative Damage Theories of Aging. Cell Metabolism. 2018 Apr 3;27(4):805-815.e4.

[7] Arbor S. Where and How in the mTOR Pathway Inhibitors Fight Aging: Rapamycin, Resveratrol, and Metformin. Resveratrol - Adding Life to Years, Not Adding Years to Life [Internet]. 2018 Nov 5 [cited 2019 Feb 6]; Available from: https://www.intechopen.com/books/resveratrol-adding-life-to-years-not-adding-years-to-life/where-and-how-in-the-mtor-pathway-inhibitors-fight-aging-rapamycin-resveratrol-and-metformin

[8] Arbor S. Targeting amyloid precursor protein shuttling and processing - long before amyloid beta formation. Neural Regen Res. 2017 Mar 7;12(2):207-209.

[9] Mirzaei H, Raynes R, Longo VD. The conserved role of protein restriction in aging and disease: Current Opinion in Clinical Nutrition and Metabolic Care. 2016 Jan;19(1):74-79.

[10] Flanagan EW, Most J, Mey JT, Redman LM. Calorie Restriction and Aging in Humans. Annu Rev Nutr. 2020 Sep 23;40(1):105-133.

[11] O'Flanagan CH, Smith LA, McDonell SB, Hursting SD. When less may be more: calorie restriction and response to cancer therapy. BMC Med [Internet]. 2017 May 24 [cited 2018 Aug 23];15. Available from: https://www.ncbi.nlm.nih.gov/pmc/articles/PMC5442682/

[12] Longo VD, Antebi A, Bartke A, Barzilai N, Brown-Borg HM, Caruso C, et al. Interventions to Slow Aging in Humans: Are We Ready? Aging Cell. 2015 Aug;14(4):497-510.

[13] Singhal S, Rosen E, Newman E, Autran L, Sam K, Rao N, et al. McKinsey on Healthcare: Best of 2019 [Internet]. McKinsey & Company; 2019 [cited 2020 Nov 16]. Available from: https://www.mckinsey.com/industries/healthcare-systems-and-services/our-insights/mckinsey-on-healthcare-best-of-2019

[14] Catillon M, Cutler DM, Getzen TE. Two hundred years of health and medical care [Internet]. VoxEU.org. 2019 [cited 2020 Nov 24]. Available from: https://voxeu.org/article/

two-hundred-years-health-and-medical-care

[15] Zeckhauser R, Shepard D. Where Now for Saving Lives? Law and Contemporary Problems. 1976 Oct 1;40(4):5-45.

[16] Pliskin JS, Shepard DS, Weinstein MC. Utility Functions for Life Years and Health Status. Operations Research. 1980;28(1):206-224.

[17] Bleichrodt H, Johannesson M. The validity of QALYs: an experimental test of constant proportional tradeoff and utility independence. Med Decis Making. 1997 Mar;17(1):21-32.

[18] Gerard K. Cost-utility in practice: a policy maker's guide to the state of the art. Health Policy. 1992 Jul;21(3): 249-279.

[19] Shepard DS. Cost-effectiveness in Health and Medicine. By M.R. Gold, J.E Siegel, L.B. Russell, and M.C. Weinstein (eds). New York: Oxford University Press, 1996. The Journal of Mental Health Policy and Economics. 1999;2(2): 91-92.

[20] Russell LB, Gold MR, Siegel JE, Daniels N, Weinstein MC. The role of cost-effectiveness analysis in health and medicine. Panel on Cost-Effectiveness in Health and Medicine. JAMA. 1996 Oct 9;276(14):1172-1177.

[21] Adamiak G. Methods for the economic evaluation of health care programmes, 3rd ed. J Epidemiol Community Health. 2006 Sep;60(9): 822-823.

[22] Torrance GW. Measurement of health state utilities for economic appraisal. J Health Econ. 1986 Mar;5(1):1-30.

[23] Jonsen AR. Bentham in a box: technology assessment and health care allocation. Law Med Health Care. 1986 Sep;14(3-4):172-174.

[24] Commissioner O of the. FDA Approves First Cell-Based Gene Therapy For Adult Patients with Relapsed or Refractory MCL [Internet]. FDA. FDA; 2020 [cited 2020 Dec 10]. Available from: https://www.fda.gov/news-events/press-announcements/fda-approves-first-cell-based-gene-therapy-adult-patients-relapsed-or-refractory-mcl

[25] Sarkar RR, Gloude NJ, Schiff D, Murphy JD. Cost-Effectiveness of Chimeric Antigen Receptor T-Cell Therapy in Pediatric Relapsed/Refractory B-Cell Acute Lymphoblastic Leukemia. J Natl Cancer Inst. 2019 01;111(7):719-26.

[26] Lin JK, Muffly LS, Spinner MA, Barnes JI, Owens DK, Goldhaber-Fiebert JD. Cost Effectiveness of Chimeric Antigen Receptor T-Cell Therapy in Multiply Relapsed or Refractory Adult Large B-Cell Lymphoma. J Clin Oncol. 2019 20;37(24):2105-19.

[27] Silbert S, Yanik GA, Shuman AG. How Should We Determine the Value of CAR T-Cell Therapy? AMA Journal of Ethics. 2019 Oct 1;21(10):844-851.

[28] McKie J, Richardson J. The rule of rescue. Soc Sci Med. 2003 Jun;56(12): 2407-2419.

[29] Ashcroft RE. Quality of Life as the Basis of Health Care Resource Allocation: A Philosopher's Perspective on QALYs. AMA Journal of Ethics. 2005 Feb 1;7(2):195-199.

[30] How Organ Donation Works | Organ Donor [Internet]. 2018 [cited 2020 Dec 13]. Available from: https://www.organdonor.gov/about/process.html

[31] Vos R, Vusser KD, Schaevers V, Schoonis A, Lemaigre V, Dobbels F, et al.

Smoking resumption after lung transplantation: a sobering truth. European Respiratory Journal. 2010 Jun 1;35(6):1411-1413.

[32] Li Y, Pan A, Wang DD, Liu X, Dhana K, Franco OH, et al. Impact of Healthy Lifestyle Factors on Life Expectancies in the US Population. Circulation. 2018 Apr 30; CIRCULATIONAHA.117.032047.

[33] Muller RA, Muller EA. Air Pollution and Cigarette Equivalence [Internet]. Berkeley Earth. [cited 2020 Dec 13]. Available from: http://berkeleyearth.org/archive/air-pollution-and-cigarette-equivalence/

[34] Rohde RA, Muller RA. Air Pollution in China: Mapping of Concentrations and Sources. PLOS ONE. 2015 Aug 20;10(8):e0135749.

[35] Tsochatzis E, Bosch J, Burroughs A. Liver cirrhosis - The Lancet. 2014 May 17;383(9930):1749-1761.

[36] Cummings J, Lee G, Ritter A, Sabbagh M, Zhong K. Alzheimer's disease drug development pipeline: 2020. Alzheimers Dement (N Y). 2020;6(1):e12050.

[37] Reitz C, Brayne C, Mayeux R. Epidemiology of Alzheimer disease. Nat Rev Neurol. 2011 Mar;7(3):137-152.

[38] Bauzon J, Lee G, Cummings J. Repurposed agents in the Alzheimer's disease drug development pipeline. Alzheimers Res Ther. 2020 Aug 17;12(1):98.

[39] Chen Z, McCulloch CE, Powe NR, Heung M, Saran R, Pavkov ME, et al. Exploring reasons for state-level variation in incidence of dialysis-requiring acute kidney injury (AKI-D) in the United States. BMC Nephrol. 2020 Aug 10;21(1):336.

[40] Chen H-Y, Kuo S, Su P-F, Wu J-S, Ou H-T. Health Care Costs Associated With Macrovascular, Microvascular, and Metabolic Complications of Type 2 Diabetes Across Time: Estimates From a Population-Based Cohort of More Than 0.8 Million Individuals With Up to 15 Years of Follow-up. Diabetes Care. 2020 Aug 1;43(8):1732-1740.

[41] The Worldview Upgrader – Gapminder launches a groundbreaking new service to fight misconceptions [Internet]. [cited 2020 Dec 14]. Available from: https://www.gapminder.org/news/the-worldview-upgrader-gapminder-launches-a-groundbreaking-new-service-to-fight-misconceptions/

[42] Rosling H, Zhang Z. Health advocacy with Gapminder animated statistics. J Epidemiol Glob Health. 2011 Dec;1(1):11-14.

[43] Lenton TM, Held H, Kriegler E, Hall JW, Lucht W, Rahmstorf S, et al. Tipping elements in the Earth's climate system. Proc Natl Acad Sci U S A. 2008 Feb 12;105(6):1786-1793.

[44] Patz JA, Olson SH. Climate change and health: global to local influences on disease risk. Ann Trop Med Parasitol. 2006 Sep;100(5-6):535-549.

[45] Schneider T, Kaul CM, Pressel KG. Possible climate transitions from breakup of stratocumulus decks under greenhouse warming. Nature Geoscience. 2019 Mar;12(3):163-167.

[46] Pal JS, Eltahir EAB. Future temperature in southwest Asia projected to exceed a threshold for human adaptability. Nature Climate Change. 2016 Feb;6(2):197-200.

[47] Im E-S, Pal JS, Eltahir EAB. Deadly heat waves projected in the densely populated agricultural regions of South Asia. Science Advances. 2017 Aug 1;3(8):e1603322.

[48] Coffel ED, Horton RM, Sherbinin A de. Temperature and humidity based projections of a rapid rise in global heat stress exposure during the 21st century. Environ Res Lett. 2017 Dec;13(1): 014001.

[49] Raymond C, Matthews T, Horton RM. The emergence of heat and humidity too severe for human tolerance. Science Advances. 2020 May 1;6(19):eaaw1838.

[50] Khan SU, Khan MZ, Alkhouli M. Trends of Clinical Outcomes and Health Care Resource Use in Heart Failure in the United States. J Am Heart Assoc. 2020 Jul 21;9(14):e016782.

[51] Osterman M, Martin J. Trends in low-risk cesarean delivery in the United States, 1990-2013 [Internet]. National Center for Health Statistics; 2014 p. 16. Available from: https://www.cdc.gov/nchs/data/nvsr/nvsr63/nvsr63_06.pdf

[52] Kuhlmann PK, Patel DN, Chen A, Houman J, Weinberger J, Wood Thum LN, et al. Economic evaluation of elective cesarean versus vaginal delivery on cost of future pelvic floor disorders in the United States. Neurourol Urodyn. 2020 Nov 24;

Section 2

Assessing Quality of Life in States of Chronic Diseases and Psychological Health

Chapter 3

Assessment of Pain, Acceptance of Illness, Adjustment to Life and Strategies of Coping with the Illness in Patients with Pancreatic Cancer

Urszula Religioni, Aleksandra Czerw,
Anna M. Badowska-Kozakiewicz, Michał Budzik
and Andrzej Deptała

Abstract

Pancreatic cancer is the fourth most common cancer causing death in the world. The prognosis of patients with pancreatic cancer is relatively low, which may be reflected in the patients' lack of acceptance of the illness and passive attitudes towards the illness. The aim of the study was to evaluate the strategy of coping with pain and its control, acceptance of the illness and adjustment to life with cancer in patients suffering from pancreatic cancer. Forty six patients with pancreatic cancer were included in the study. They were treated as outpatients at the Center of Oncology at Maria Skłodowska-Curie's Institute in Warsaw between 2017 and 2018. The questionnaire included four psychometric tests: BPCQ, CSQ, AIS and MiniMAC. In the BPCQ test the highest average test result was obtained by "internal factors" (M = 16.85; SD = 5.64). The most frequently chosen strategies for coping with pain are praying/hoping (M = 22.33; SD = 7.85). The average illness acceptance score was 23.13 (SD = 7.84). The most common methods of psychological adjustment to cancer for the studied group are the strategies of positive re-evaluation (M = 20.07, SD = 3.67). Patients with pancreatic cancer have a low level of acceptance of their illness.

Keywords: pancreatic cancer, pain control, coping with pain, acceptance of illness

1. Introduction

According to data available in the National Cancer Registry, the number of pancreatic cancers in Poland in 2016 was over 3,486 (standardized ratio 5.5/100,000). In 2016, pancreatic cancer in the illness mortality structure in Poland took eighth place in men (2.1%) and eleventh in women (2.1%). Most pancreatic cancers are diagnosed in Poland after the age of 50 [1, 2].

In Poland, pancreatic cancer occurs less frequently than in most European Union countries. Pancreatic cancer is much more common in developed countries (North

America, Central and Northern Europe, Australia) than in African or Indian countries. The American statistical data from 2018 provided the number of 56,770 new cases, including 29,940 in men and 26,830 in women (fourth place in the mortality structure in men and women) [3].

Pancreatic cancer is the fourth most common cancer causing death in the world [4]. In Poland, it is the sixth most common cause of deaths for men (4.3% in the mortality structure) and five women (5.6% in the mortality structure) due to cancer. In 2016, a total of 4,908 Poles died due to pancreatic cancer (standardized ratio 6.2/100,000), and this ratio is comparable to the average of the European Union countries and other countries in the world. The 5-year survival rate in patients with pancreatic cancer in Poland is 9.0% [1, 2].

Risk factors for pancreatic cancer include genetic factors, smoking, obesity, diet rich in red meat and animal fats, and chronic pancreatitis. Surgical treatment is the only method that allows complete cure of pancreatic cancer, provided there is no metastasis at the time of diagnosis, however, due to significant illness severity, only 15–20% of patients can be optimally treated surgically [5].

Due to the very low survival rate of patients with pancreatic cancer (on average 3–7 months from diagnosis and 10–15% one year), it is important that the treatment of patients takes into account the achievement of the highest quality of life [6, 7]. The subjectively assessed quality of life of patients with cancer largely depends on the acceptance of cancer and coping with pain and illness. In the case of pancreatic cancer, patients, having knowledge that survival with this type of illness is very low, may have a tendency to choose destructive behaviors in coping with the illness, which may affect the quality of life they assess, increase pain, and affect the effects of treatment.

The aim of the study was to assess the level of acceptance of the illness, strategies for coping with pain, locating pain control, as well as adapting to life with cancer in patients with pancreatic cancer. The study looked for relationships between socio-economic factors (sex, age, education, professional status, income, place of residence) and treatment with chemotherapy, and results obtained in psychometric tests.

2. Material and methods

The study was conducted between 2017 and mid-2018 among 46 patients diagnosed with pancreatic cancer in stage II-IV according to the AJCC 2017, 8th ed. The outpatients were treated with chemotherapy with gemcitabine at the Center of Oncology at Maria Sklodowska-Curie's Institute in Warsaw. The study tool was a questionnaire with metric questions and four psychometric tests:

1. The Beliefs about Pain Control Questionnaire (BPCQ), designed to examine people suffering from pain.

2. The Pain Coping Strategies Questionnaire (CSQ), used to examine people who complain about pain.

3. Approval Illness Scale (AIS), measuring the level of adjustment to the illness.

4. Mental Adjustment to Cancer Scale (Mini-MAC), measuring the level of mental adjustment to cancer.

The PAPI (Paper and Pencil Interview) technique was used in the study. All patients included in the study gave consented to carry it out.

The study findings were then statistically analyzed with the use of Student's t-test for independent samples, one-way analysis of variance and Pearson's r correlation (in the case of age variable). The adopted statistical significance was at $p < 0.05$.

The scores of the tests were correlated with socioeconomic characteristics of the respondents: sex, age, education, professional status, place of residence, net income-per-household-member, and with chemotherapy treatment in the past year.

3. Results

The study involved patients aged 30–84 years (M = 60.46, SD = 12.28), including 24 (52.2%) women aged 43–84 (M = 63.71, SD = 12.08) and 22 (47.8%) men aged 30–74 (M = 56.91, SD = 11.74).

Among the studied group of patients, 16 (34.8%) have primary/vocational education, 14 (30.4%) have secondary, and 16 (34.8%) have higher education. Over half of the patients - 26 (56.5%) live in towns with a population of up to 100,000, and 20 (43.5%) live in cities with a population of over 100,000. Half of the patients have a monthly net income of up to PLN 1,500 (23 patients, 50.0%), thereby 50% patients indicated that they achieved income over PLN 1,500.00. There were 20 people (43.5%) working in the examined group, and 26 patients (56.5%) were pensioners (56.5%).

In 23 patients (50.0%) metastases were diagnosed. Among the studied group of patients, 25 (54.3%) were undergoing chemotherapy treatment, 15 (32.6%) were undergoing radiotherapy and 10 subjects (21.7%) were undergoing targeted treatment.

3.1 Pain control

In the assessment of pain control in patients with pancreatic cancer S. Skevington's BPCQ (The Beliefs about Pain Control Questionnaire), consisting of 13 statements, was used. In accordance with the assumptions of the BPCQ, the statements used in the questionnaire constitute a part of three factors that measure the strength of individual beliefs about controlling pain personally (internal factors), influence of physicians (other forces), or by random events [8].

In the case of patients with pancreatic cancer, the highest average score in the BPCQ questionnaire was obtained by "internal factors" (M = 16.85; SD = 5.64), and the lowest – "random events" (M = 14.85; SD = 4.11) (**Table 1**), which means that patients believe that these factors contribute to pain control.

Socio-economic variables that differentiate results in patients with pancreatic cancer are gender and net income per household member. In the case of gender, there was a statistically significant difference in the internal locus of pain control ($p = 0.024$). The mean value obtained in the group of women (M = 18.63) was higher than in the group of men (M = 14.91).

The level of income in the studied group of patients influenced the difference in the locus of pain control in random events ($p = 0.027$). The mean value of the severity of the locus of pain control in random events was higher in the group of people with higher income above PLN 1,500 (M = 16.17) than in those in the case of whom in the household the income per family member does not exceed PLN 1,500 (M = 13.52).

Other variables (age, education, place of residence, professional status and chemotherapy) did not affect the results of the pain control questionnaire.

3.2 Pain coping strategies

The Pain Coping Strategies Questionnaire developed by A.K. Rosenstiel and F.J. Keefe (CSQ) is used to examine people who complain about pain. The questionnaire consists of 42 statements and is intended to assess the pain coping strategies that patients use, as well as to verify the effectiveness of these strategies in reducing or managing pain. The ways of dealing with pain assessed in the questionnaire reflect six cognitive and one behavioral strategy, which in turn constitute a part of three factors: cognitive coping, distracting and taking substitute actions, and catastrophizing and seeking hope [9].

In the BPCQ the highest average score for respondents suffering from pancreatic cancer was obtained by praying/hoping (M = 22.33; SD = 7.85), then declaring coping (M = 19.83; SD = 8.06) and increased behavioral activity (M = 19.67; SD = 8.59). According to patients, these factors have the greatest impact on the fight against cancer. The smallest values are visible in the case of re-evaluation of pain (M = 13.35; SD = 9.24) and ignoring sensations (M = 14.93; SD = 9.36) (**Figure 1**).

The assessment that was particularly differentiated by the socio-economic variables under study is praying/hoping. The results in this assessment are differentiated by gender, age, occupational status and the fact that patients have undergone chemotherapeutic treatment in the last year.

In the case of gender, it was noticed that the average value of the praying/hoping assessment was significantly higher in the group of women than men (p = 0.030), and the average values of this assessment were 24.71 for women and 19.73 for men respectively.

In the assessment of praying/hoping, statistically significant positive correlations were obtained in the case of the age of the respondents (r = 0.367). In addition, the age of patients positively correlated with the assessment of increased behavioral activity (r = 0.387).

The average value of the praying/hoping dimension was also higher in the group of pensioners than in the group of working patients (p = 0.044), amounting to 24.48 for pensioners and 19.75 for working people.

Patients who have not been subjected to chemotherapy in the last year also had a higher average value of praying/hoping in the BPCQ (M = 25.52) than patients who were subjected to chemotherapy (M = 19.64) (p = 0.010).

Patients' education, place of residence and income per family member did not affect the pain coping strategies adopted by patients.

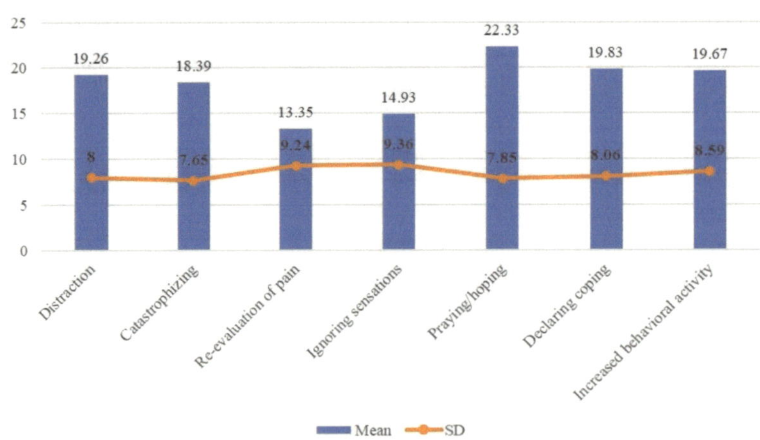

Figure 1.
Results of the CSQ for patients with pancreatic cancer.

3.3 Acceptance of illness

The Approval Illness Scale (AIS) consists of eight statements, based on which the results obtainable for each respondent in the level of acceptance of the illness are within the range from 8 to 40. The higher the score, the better adjustment to the illness and the lesser the sense of mental discomfort. The lower the score, the greater the severity of negative emotions associated with the illness, and thus its lower acceptance [10].

The mean score (disease acceptance level) obtained by patients suffering from pancreatic cancer in the AIS scale was 23.13 with a standard deviation of 7.84. None of the socio-economic variables studied determines differences in the level of illness acceptance between groups.

The average value of acceptance of the illness in the group of women was 22.54 and was close to the average value obtained in the group of men, which was 23.77. The average value of acceptance of the illness in the group of people with primary or vocational education was 22.08, in the group of people with secondary education was 23.43, and in the group of people with higher education was 23.13.

The average disease acceptance was similar in the group of people living in towns with a population of up to 100,000, and in towns with a population above 100,000 (23.1 and 23.15, respectively).Income also did not differentiate the obtained results. The average value of acceptance of the illness in the group of people with net income of up to PLN 1,500 per person in the family was 23.61 and was also close to the average value obtained in the group of people who achieved income above PLN 1,500 ($M = 22.65$).

The average value of acceptance of the illness in the working group was 24.85, and in the group of pensioners - 21.52, but these differences were also not statistically significant.

The average value of acceptance of the illness in the group of patients who underwent the chemotherapeutic treatment last year was 22.84 and similarly to other variables it was close to the average value obtained in the group of people who did not undergo chemotherapy treatment which was 23.48.

3.4 Mental adjustment to the illness

The Mini-Mac (Mental Adjustment to Cancer) questionnaire measures four methods of mental adjustment to the illness: anxiety, fighting spirit, helplessness - hopelessness and positive reevaluation. According to the assumptions of the questionnaire, anxiety and helplessness-hopelessness are part of a passive (destructive) style of coping with the illness, and the other two dimensions refer to the active (constructive) style of coping with the illness [11].

Respondents suffering from pancreatic cancer obtained the highest result of the Mini-Mac test in terms of positive re-evaluation ($M = 20.07$, $SD = 3.67$) and fighting spirit ($M = 19.80$, $SD = 3.89$) and these are the main disease adaptation methods used by patients, and the lowest - in terms of helplessness-hopelessness ($M = 15.87$, $SD = 4.56$) (**Table 2**).

The strategy of positive re-evaluation was differentiated by the gender of patients ($p = 0.002$). The average value of positive re-evaluation obtained in the group of women was higher than in the group of men (respectively $M = 21.63$ and $M = 18.36$). Similarly, the average in positive re-evaluation was dependent on the age of patients - the higher the age, the higher the values obtained by patients in this assessment ($r = 0.550$). The age of the patients also positively correlated with fighting spirit ($r = 0.429$).

The average value of positive re-evaluation was statistically significantly lower in the group of patients with higher education ($M = 17.50$) than in the group with basic or vocational education (M = 21.00) and in the group of people with secondary education (M = 21.93) (p = 0.001).

Income also conditioned the value of positive re-evaluation (p = 0.004). The average value of positive re-evaluation was higher in the group of people with lower income up to PLN 1,500 per person in the family (M = 21.57) in comparison with people whose income per family member exceeded PLN 1,500 (M = 18.57).

Positive re-evaluation was also conditioned by the professional status of patients (p = 0.001). The average value of this assessment was higher in the group of pensioners (M = 21.83) than in the group of working patients (M = 17.70).

4. Discussion

Chronic illness forces patients to make many changes in their life to be able to adapt to the new situation. In this area, accepting the losses caused by the illness seems to be the most difficult for patients, coping with the limitations and measuring the risks that may arise in connection with cancer [12].

Pancreatic cancer is usually diagnosed at an advanced stage, which results from the fact that the patient feels the symptoms only when the illness is fully developed and the metastases are already distant. At the same time, late diagnosis of the illness is associated with rapidly developing, difficult to treat symptoms, which in the case of pancreatic cancer include quick destruction of the body, lack of appetite, pain, pruritus, nausea and vomiting, deep vein thrombosis. Many patients with pancreatic cancer do not survive the first year after the diagnosis, and with severe pain and high severity of cancer symptoms it seems reasonable to implement palliative care in the first months after the diagnosis [13]. Furthermore, patients themselves are aware that the survival rate with pancreatic cancer is one of the lowest of all cancers, which is additionally a stress factor for patients.

A study to assess the level of stress and depression among patients with various cancers indicates that patients with pancreatic cancer are most affected by anxiety and are characterized by the highest rate of depression [14, 15]. Similar results are indicated by Clark K.L. et al. [16].

Many studies indicate that subjective feelings, attitudes and behaviors influence pain. Pain as a physical and psychological phenomenon is felt with the participation of consciousness, therefore the state of the psyche and psychological factors play a fundamental role in experiencing pain, especially chronic pain. Particularly important element affecting the experience of pain is the control locus (locus of control is the degree to which people believe they control the situations they experience in lives; control can be internal or external) which also directly affects the behavior of the patient in a situation of pain [17–19].

Our study, including 46 patients with pancreatic cancer, indicates that patients control pain mainly through internal factors (M = 16.85, SD = 5.64). A similar result is obtained by patients with cancer of the digestive system - colorectal cancer (N = 238; M = 17.36; SD = 5.48) [20]. Studies conducted by Basińska M.A. et al. also using the BPCQ questionnaire in patients with colorectal cancer and lung cancer indicate that in both groups the patients attribute the greatest role in the control of pain to the influence of physicians (for patients with lung cancer M = 17.08, SD 4.97, and for patients with colorectal cancer M = 16.98, SD = 4.32) (**Table 3**). Patients attribute the lowest role of pain control to random events (for patients with lung cancer M = 15.18, SD = 3.80, and for patients with colorectal cancer M = 15.00, SD = 3.46), and these values are very similar to the sense of control through internal factors. The study conducted by Basińska M.A. et al. at the same time, indicated that patients with external control locus use methods of passively struggling with the illness and vice versa - patients with high internal control locus are characterized by high activity and better psychological well-being. The external health control locus is associated with chronic negative emotions such as depression, anxiety or hostility, as well as an increase in pain symptoms in patients [17].

According to our study, the most common way to cope with pain in the case of patients with pancreatic cancer is praying/hoping (M = 22.33, SD = 7.85), typical primarily for women, the elderly, and pensioners. These groups obtained by far the highest values in the assessment of praying/hoping. Patients with colorectal cancer in the study conducted by Czerw A. et al. most often use coping strategies and increased behavioral activity [20] also typical for prostate cancer [21], lung cancer [22] and breast cancer [23] (**Figure 2**). Interestingly, among patients with colorectal cancer, it was noticed that the strategy of praying/hoping is particularly often chosen by women and the group of pensioners [20], as in the case of patients with pancreatic cancer according to our study.

The strategies of praying/hoping and declaring coping typical for patients with pancreatic cancer are the most commonly used in the group of patients chronically ill with back pain in the studies conducted by A.K. Rosenstiel and F.J. Keefe. Similarly, the most rarely used strategy for patients was the re-evaluation of pain [9], and this assessment was also poorly assessed by patients in our study. Although, Religioni U. et al. [24] in the study conducted on cancer patients indicates that socio-economic variables, which most often differentiate the selection of strategies for coping with cancer pain, are education and income, in the case of patients with pancreatic cancer, this relationship was not noticed.

However, it should be noted that many studies indicate that the strategies of catastrophizing or praying/hoping significantly affect the severity of pain symptoms in chronic illnesses and deterioration of the general health condition [25, 26].

The level of acceptance of the illness among patients with pancreatic cancer in our study was 23.13 (SD = 7.84). The acceptance of the illness in the studied group is lower than in the group of patients with other cancers (among patients with breast cancer the average disease acceptance score in the AIS test was 28.46, among patients with lung cancer M = 23.17, among patients with cancer of the large intestine M = 27.74, among prostate cancer patients M = 30.39) [27]. Similarly,

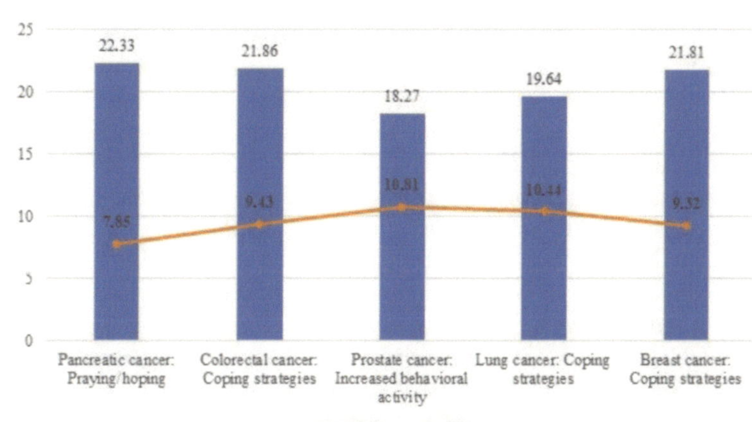

Figure 2.
The most common way to cope with pain in cancer patients [20–23].

Kapela I. et al. indicate that among patients with colorectal cancer, the level of acceptance of the disease according to the AIS scale reaches values slightly higher than the average (M = 28.4) and close to the values obtained in the studies conducted by Religioni U. et al. [28].

Significantly lower results in the AIS test were obtained by Kozak G. Among the oncological patients subject to palliative care, the highest level of acceptance of the illness was observed in women with cancer of the reproductive organs (M = 21.93, SD = 6.00) compared to patients with colorectal cancer (M = 16.58, SD = 7.42), gastric cancer (M = 16.87, SD = 5.59) and pancreatic cancer (M = 18.23, SD = 9.13) [29]. The level of acceptance of the illness in patients with various cancers, including pancreatic cancer, examined by Kołpa M. et al. was on average M = 25.35; SD = 9.25. This study indicates that age diversifies the level of adjustment to the illness, but other variables, such as education or gender, do not affect the results [30]. In the study of patients with pancreatic cancer none of the variables affected the level of acceptance of the illness.

The study conducted on other groups of patients indicates that such patients get higher results in the AIS test than patients with pancreatic cancer, e.g. patients with diabetes M = 25.76; SD = 10.34, patients with cardiovascular disease M = 27.78; SD = 9.86, patients with diseases of the nervous system M = 27.02; SD = 8.92 [12].

Among the available studies only few groups achieve lower values in the AIS test compared to patients with pancreatic cancer in our study: men after myocardial infarction (M = 22.14), men with chronic pain (M = 18.44), men with back pain (M = 20.51) [31].

The level of disease acceptance among patients with various types of cancer is presented in **Table 4**.

Pancreatic cancer is a specific type of cancer. The coping process is dynamic and involves various strategies, the use of which depends on the duration of the illness [32]. Among the methods of coping with cancer by patients with pancreatic cancer, positive re-evaluation (M = 20.07, SD = 3.67) and fighting spirit (M = 19,8; SD = 3,89) dominate. In patients with colorectal cancer in the study conducted by Kapela I. et al. the constructive style dominates as well, with a predominance of fighting spirit (M = 23.9) and positive re-evaluation (M = 22.5) [28]. Similar results were obtained by Czerw A. et al. among patients with colorectal cancer (fighting spirit M = 23.42, positive re-evaluation M = 22.31) [20].

The average results for anxiety and hopelessness/hopelessness in our study were respectively M = 18.30;SD = 4.72 and M = 15.87; SD = 4.56, which is a much higher result than in the case of other most common cancers (lung, breast, colon and prostate cancer) [33]. Similar, although higher results for these assessments are indicated by Kozak G. In his studies, men with prostate cancer have the highest intensity of anxiety among all cancer patients. Anxiety is also significantly higher in the case of patients with stomach cancer (M = 22.84; SD = 5.52), pancreas cancer (M = 22.43; SD = 6.30) and colorectal cancer (M = 21.72; SD = 6.55) in comparison to women with cancer of the reproductive organs (M = 18.34; SD = 4.26). In the case of these patients, the highest level of fighting spirit is observed (M = 23.95; SD = 4.35). In the studies conducted by Kozak G. a significantly higher level of fighting spirit was observed in patients with stomach cancer (M = 19.62; SD = 5.82) and colorectal cancer (M = 19.37; SD = 5.32) in comparison to patients with pancreatic cancer M = 15.43; SD = 5.01) or prostate cancer (M = 15.68; SD = 5.06). Patients with stomach cancer (M = 20.98; SD = 5.68), pancreatic cancer (M = 21.22; SD = 5.10) and colorectal cancer (M = 19.16; SD = 7.41) are characterized by greater severity of helplessness/hopelessness compared to women with cancer of the reproductive organs (M = 13.70; SD = 5.36) (**Table 5**) [29].

The analysis of the level of acceptance of the illness in relation to the adopted way of adjustment to the illness indicated that the higher the level of acceptance on the AIS scale, the higher the level of fighting spirit and the level on the scale of the constructive style (Mini-MAC) [30]. In this context, the implementation of activities aimed at helping to accept the disease is particularly important. These actions should be taken by medical personnel. Health policy programs can also play an important role in this respect. These programs may include specialist trainings for medical personnel as well as implementation of activities directed directly to patients [34].

Similarly, in the study conducted on 220 patients with various cancers: stomach cancer, cancer of reproductive organs, pancreatic cancer, colorectal cancer and prostate cancer, similar dependencies were indicated – the higher the acceptance of the illness, the higher the intensity of fighting spirit and the lower the intensity of anxiety and helplessness/hopelessness [29]. In the study conducted on patients with colorectal patients, education significantly affects the results obtained in terms of anxiety, helplessness/hopelessness and the destructive style [28]. In our study conducted on patients with pancreatic cancer, education positively correlated with the strategy of positive re-evaluation. Among patients with pancreatic cancer in the study conducted by Kozak G., it was also observed that the older the patients, the lower the intensity of anxiety and helplessness/hopelessness [29]. A similar relationship in this group of patients was also described by Juczyński Z., although our study does not confirm this dependency. Numerous studies indicate that a typical method to cope with the illness among patients with pancreatic cancer is the application of defense mechanisms – repression and denial. According to Bahnson C. et al., repression and denial play a key role in the development of cancer, including pancreatic cancer [35, 36].

As authors, we are aware of the imitations of our research. First of all, we know that our sample of patients is small. The study took place in an outpatient clinic, and we recruited as many patients as possible. However, we know that extending the study to include hospitalized patients would bring more accurate results. We believe that this is the direction of further research. Additionally, despite identifying the benefits of some psychological strategies, we recognize that our research only shows the course of action. It is not possible to force a patient to adopt any disease strategy. This attitude must result from their internal needs and beliefs. However, the skillful help of a psychologist can help patients fight the disease so that the patient experiences the highest possible quality of life.

5. Conclusions

1. Patients with pancreatic cancer assign the greatest role in the locus of pain control to internal factors.

2. Dominant strategies for coping with pain by the studied patients involve praying/hoping and declaring coping, especially in the group of women, the elderly, and pensioners and people who have not undergone chemotherapy in the last year.

3. Patients suffering from pancreatic cancer have a relatively low level of acceptance of their illness, and this result is not dependent on the socio-economic variables studied.

4. Patients with pancreatic cancer usually have a constructive style of coping with the illness, although anxiety and helplessness/hopelessness in the case of these patients also obtain rather high values.

5. The study of patients' quality of life, including the level of acceptance of the illness or styles of coping with the illness is particularly important among people with pancreatic cancer. These studies should become one of the elements of comprehensive oncological care, in which the process of treating patients should also include psychological care.

Conflict of interest

None declared.

Declarations

Ethics approval and consent to participate

Ethics Committee of the Medical University of Warsaw approved this study. Due to the scope of the data, we obtained verbal informed consent.

A. Appendix

A.1 Statistical analysis of the results

A.1.1 Descriptive statistics

Table 1 presents descriptive statistics for the analyzed variables, i.e. mean values, standard deviations as well as minimum and maximum results. The list was also supplemented with the values of the Kolmogorov-Smirnov test verifying the assumption about the normality of the distribution of the analyzed variables and the values of skewness and kurtosis measures.

No statistically significant deviations from the normal distribution were obtained.

	Variable	*M.*	*SD*	*min*	*max*	*WITH*	*p*	*S.*	*K.*
Strategies	Distraction	19.26	8.00	2	36	0.65	0.794	4.00	−0.12
counseling	Re-evaluation of pain sensations	13.35	9.24	0	36	1.01	0.257	0.02	−0.39
myself	Catastrophizing	18.39	7.65	2	33	0.64	0.804	−0.09	−0.31
with pain	Ignoring sensations	14.93	9.36	0	36	0.61	0.844	−0.05	−0.65
	Praying/Hope	22.33	7.85	9	36	0.72	0.673	0.09	−1.04
	Declaring coping	19.83	8.06	7	36	0.91	0.374	0.20	−0.99
	Increased behavioral activity	19.67	8.59	2	36	0.63	0.819	0.14	−0.61
Adaptation	Anxiety preoccupation	18.30	4.72	8	28	0.60	0.865	0.04	−0.52
mental	Fighting spirit	19.80	3.89	9	28	0.59	0.882	0.04	0.55
to disease	Helplessness-hopelessness	15.87	4.56	7	26	0.66	0.776	0.11	−0.65

	Variable	M.	SD	min	max	WITH	p	S.	K.
cancerous	Positive reevaluation	20.07	3.67	12	28	0.78	0.584	−0.28	−0.34
	Acceptance of the disease	23.13	7.84	8	38	0.61	0.857	−0.18	−0.84
Control	Inside	16.85	5.64	6	thirty	0.78	0.581	0.16	0.04
pain	The influence of doctors	16.54	4.21	5	24	0.59	0.875	−0.04	0.15
	Random events	14.85	4.11	7	24	0.58	0.892	0.03	−0.25

M.- average value; SD - standard deviation; min - minimum value; max - maximum value; Z - value of the Kolmogorov–Smirnov test; p - statistical significance; S - skewness measure; K - measure of kurtosis.

Table 1.
Descriptive statistics for the analyzed variables.

A.1.2 Results

A.1.2.1 Pain coping strategies

Based on the results of the analysis of variance with repeated measures, it was found that there were statistically significant differences between the intensity of individual pain coping strategies, F (3.71; 166.97) = 9.33, $p < 0.001$, $\eta^2 = 0.17$. **Figure 3** shows the mean values of the intensity of the analyzed strategies along with the confidence intervals determined based on the Bonferroni correction.

It was found that praying/hoping was a strategy used more often than reevaluating pain sensations and ignoring sensations. Re-evaluation of pain sensations was a less frequently used strategy than distraction and catastrophizing.

Table 2 presents the mean values of the intensity of coping strategies in the group of women and men. The list was supplemented with the values of the Student's two-sided t-test for independent samples.

There was a statistically significant difference in the prayer/hope strategy.

Table 3 shows the Pearson r correlation coefficients between the age of the respondents and the coping strategies. Statistically significant correlations were marked.

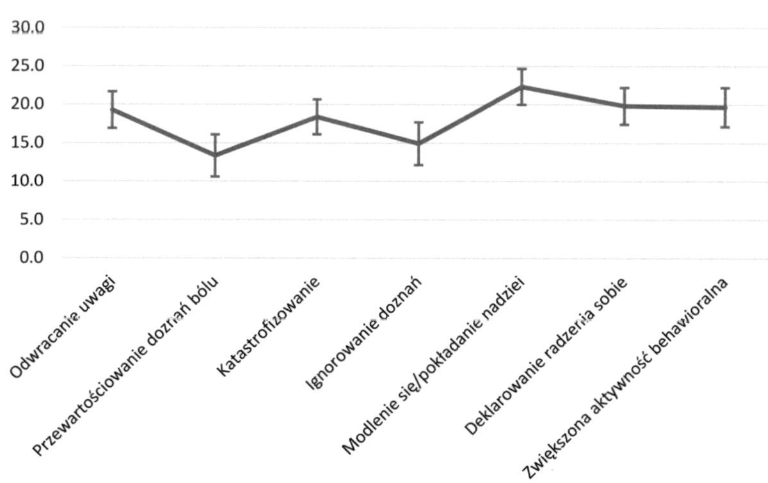

Figure 3.
The mean values of the intensity of the analyzed strategies with confidence intervals determined based on the Bonferroni correction.

	Women		Men				
Variable	***M.***	***SD***	***M.***	***SD***	***vol***	***df***	***p***
Distraction	20.71	8.72	17.68	7.01	1.29	44	0.204
Re-evaluation of pain sensations	13.33	9.67	13.36	8.97	−0.01	44	0.991
Catastrophizing	18.13	6.91	18.68	8.54	−0.24	44	0.808
Ignoring sensations	15.63	9.44	14.18	9.44	0.52	44	0.607
Praying/Hope	**24.71**	**7.90**	**19.73**	**7.09**	**2.24**	**44**	**0.030**
Declaring coping	19.88	8.78	19.77	7.40	0.04	44	0.966
Increased behavioral activity	20.79	9.78	18.45	7.10	0.92	44	0.363

M.- average value; SD - standard deviation; t - value of the Student's t-test; df - the number of degrees of freedom; p - statistical significance.

Table 2.
Mean values of the intensity of coping with pain in the group of women and in the group of men.

Variables	**Age**
Distraction	0.276
Re-evaluation of pain sensations	0.092
Catastrophizing	−0.229
Ignoring sensations	0.089
Praying/Hope	0.369*
Declaring coping	0.207
Increased behavioral activity	0.387**

$^{*}p < 0.05$.
$^{**}p < 0.01$.

Table 3.
Pearson's r correlation coefficients between the age of the respondents and the strategies of coping with pain.

Statistically significant positive correlations were found between the age of the respondents and praying/hoping and increased behavioral activity.

Table 4 shows the mean values of the strategies of coping with pain in the group of people with primary or vocational education, in the group of people with secondary education and in the group of people with higher education. The summary was supplemented with the values of one-way analysis of variance.

No statistically significant differences were obtained.

Table 5 shows the average values of pain coping strategies in the group of people living in towns with a population of up to 100,000 and in the group of people living in towns with more than 100,000 inhabitants. The list was supplemented with the values of the Student's two-sided t-test for independent samples.

There were no statistically significant differences.

Table 6 shows the average values of the pain coping strategies in the group of people with the average monthly net income per family member up to PLN 1,500 and in the group of people with the average monthly net income per family member above PLN 1,500. The list was supplemented with the values of the Student's two-sided t-test for independent samples.

There were no statistically significant differences.

	Education							
	basic/valve		**medium**		**higher**			
Variable	*M.*	*SD*	*M.*	*SD*	*M.*	*SD*	*F.*	*p*
Distraction	22.69	6.84	18.00	9.82	16.94	6.49	2.46	0.097
Re-evaluation of pain sensations	16.44	9.70	10.21	9.78	13.00	7.72	1.77	0.183
Catastrophizing	17.81	9.52	17.43	8.44	19.81	4.46	0.42	0.659
Ignoring sensations	16.81	9.74	12.93	10.13	14.81	8.46	0.63	0.535
Praying/Hope	21.06	8.93	26.36	6.99	20.06	6.38	2.95	0.063
Declaring coping	20.63	7.71	19.93	8.22	18.94	8.68	0.17	0.844
Increased behavioral activity	22.31	6.67	18.14	11.29	18.38	7.43	1.17	0.321

M.- average value; SD - standard deviation; F - value of the one-way analysis of variance; p - statistical significance.

Table 4.
Average values of the strategies of coping with pain in the group of people with primary or vocational education, in the group of people with secondary education and in the group of people with higher education.

	The number of residents						
	up to 100,000		**over 100 thousand**				
Variable	*M.*	*SD*	*M.*	*SD*	*vol*	*df*	*p*
Distraction	18.92	7.66	19.70	8.61	−0.32	44	0.748
Re-evaluation of pain sensations	14.00	10.61	12.50	7.26	0.54	44	0.591
Catastrophizing	19.12	7.95	17.45	7.33	0.73	44	0.470
Ignoring sensations	15.15	9.85	14.65	8.94	0.18	44	0.859
Praying/Hope	23.50	7.38	20.80	8.37	1.16	44	0.252
Declaring coping	19.73	7.86	19.95	8.52	−0.09	44	0.928
Increased behavioral activity	20.42	7.96	18.70	9.48	0.67	44	0.506

M.- average value; SD - standard deviation; t - value of the Student's t-test; df - the number of degrees of freedom; p - statistical significance.

Table 5.
Average values of the pain coping strategy in the group of people living in towns with a population of up to 100,000 and in the group of people living in towns with more than 100,000 inhabitants.

Table 7 presents the mean values of the strategies of coping with pain in the group of working people and in the group of retirees and pensioners. The list was supplemented with the values of Student's two-sided t-test for independent samples.

A statistically significant difference was obtained in terms of praying/hoping.

Table 8 shows the mean values of the strategies of coping with pain in the group of patients with diagnosed metastases and in the group of patients without metastases. The list was supplemented with the values of the Student's two-sided t-test for independent samples.

Statistically significant intergroup differences in catastrophizing and declaring coping were obtained.

Table 9 shows the mean values of the pain coping strategies in the group of people who were undergoing chemotherapy and those who were not undergoing chemotherapy. The list was supplemented with the values of the Student's two-sided t-test for independent samples.

	Average monthly net income						
	up to PLN 1,500		over 1500 zlotys				
Variable	*M.*	*SD*	*M.*	*SD*	*vol*	*df*	*p*
Distraction	19.09	8.84	19.43	7.27	−0.15	44	0.885
Re-evaluation of pain sensations	12.83	8.89	13.87	9.75	−0.38	44	0.706
Catastrophizing	18.22	8.13	18.57	7.32	−0.15	44	0.879
Ignoring sensations	12.91	8.33	16.96	10.07	−1.48	44	0.145
Praying/Hope	24.17	7.99	20.48	7.43	1.62	44	0.111
Declaring coping	18.87	6.88	20.78	9.15	−0.80	44	0.427
Increased behavioral activity	18.83	8.32	20.52	8.96	−0.66	44	0.510

M.- average value; SD - standard deviation; t - value of the Student's t-test; df - the number of degrees of freedom; p - statistical significance.

Table 6.
Average values of the pain coping strategy in the group of people with an average monthly net income per family member up to PLN 1,500 and in the group of people with an average monthly net income per family member above PLN 1,500.

	Professional status						
	working		retirees/pensioners				
Variable	*M.*	*SD*	*M.*	*SD*	*vol*	*df*	*p*
Distraction	17.50	7.69	20.96	7.92	−1.45	41	0.155
Re-evaluation of pain sensations	12.80	8.32	12.96	10.35	−0.05	41	0.957
Catastrophizing	17.65	6.12	18.43	8.76	−0.34	41	0.739
Ignoring sensations	15.20	7.70	14.43	10.94	0.26	41	0.795
Praying/Hope	**19.75**	**6.46**	**24.48**	**8.21**	**−2.07**	**41**	**0.044**
Declaring coping	20.30	7.44	19.87	8.95	0.17	41	0.866
Increased behavioral activity	17.20	6.69	21.65	9.45	−1.76	41	0.086

M.- average value; SD - standard deviation; t - value of the Student's t-test; df - the number of degrees of freedom; p - statistical significance.

Table 7.
Average values of strategies for coping with pain in the group of working people and in the group of retirees and pensioners.

The mean value of the level of praying/hoping was statistically significantly lower in the group of people who were undergoing chemotherapy treatment than in the group of people who were not undergoing chemotherapy.

Table 10 presents the mean values of the pain coping strategies in the group of people who were treated with radiotherapy and in the group of people who were not treated with radiotherapy. The list was supplemented with the values of the Student's two-sided t-test for independent samples.

A statistically significant difference was obtained in the level of ignoring sensations.

Table 11 shows the mean values of the strategies of coping with pain in the group of people who were undergoing targeted therapy and in the group of people

	Known metastases						
	Yes		no				
Variable	*M.*	*SD*	*M.*	*SD*	*vol*	*df*	*p*
Distraction	18.35	7.24	21.43	8.09	−1.33	42	0.190
Re-evaluation of pain sensations	12.04	8.17	15.71	10.00	−1.34	42	0.188
Catastrophizing	**20.96**	**6.65**	**15.38**	**7.51**	**2.61**	**42**	**0.012**
Ignoring sensations	15.04	9.25	15.67	9.64	−0.22	42	0.828
Praying/Hope	20.87	7.14	24.76	8.02	−1.70	42	0.096
Declaring coping	**17.09**	**6.97**	**23.71**	**7.67**	**−3.00**	**42**	**0.004**
Increased behavioral activity	18.96	7.97	21.48	8.99	−0.99	42	0.330

M.- average value; SD - standard deviation; t - value of the Student's t-test; df - the number of degrees of freedom; p - statistical significance.

Table 8.
Mean values of strategies of coping with pain in the group of people with diagnosed metastases and in the group of people without metastases.

	Chemotherapeutic treatment						
	Yes		no				
Variable	*M.*	*SD*	*M.*	*SD*	*vol*	*df*	*p*
Distraction	18.96	6.43	19.62	9.71	−0.28	44	0.784
Re-evaluation of pain sensations	12.08	8.16	14.86	10.38	−1.02	44	0.315
Catastrophizing	19.72	8.12	16.81	6.90	1.30	44	0.202
Ignoring sensations	14.40	9.10	15.57	9.86	−0.42	44	0.677
Praying/Hope	**19.64**	**6.39**	**25.52**	**8.37**	**−2.70**	**44**	**0.010**
Declaring coping	18.32	6.43	21.62	9.51	−1.35	34.12	0.185
Increased behavioral activity	18.64	7.07	20.90	10.16	−0.89	44	0.379

M.- average value; SD - standard deviation; t - value of the Student's t-test; df - the number of degrees of freedom; p - statistical significance.

Table 9.
Average values of the strategies of coping with pain in the group of people who were undergoing chemotherapy treatment and in the group of people who were not undergoing chemotherapy.

who were not undergoing targeted therapy. The list was supplemented with the values of the Student's two-sided t-test for independent samples.

Statistically significant differences between groups were obtained in terms of re-evaluation of pain sensations and of ignoring sensations.

A.1.3 Mental adjustment to neoplastic disease

Based on the results of the analysis of variance with repeated measurements, it was found that there were also statistically significant differences between the intensity of individual indicators of mental adaptation to cancer, F (1.54; 69.45) = 9.37, $p < 0.01$, $\eta^2 = 0.17$. **Figure 4** shows the mean values of the intensity of the analyzed fitness indices together with the confidence intervals determined based on the Bonferroni correction.

Treatment with radiation therapy							
	Yes		no				
Variable	*M.*	*SD*	*M.*	*SD*	*vol*	*df*	*p*
Distraction	20.07	7.41	18.87	8.37	0.47	44	0.640
Re-evaluation of pain sensations	15.87	5.63	12.13	10.42	1.58	43.33	0.122
Catastrophizing	18.07	6.84	18.55	8.12	−0.20	44	0.844
Ignoring sensations	**19.07**	**6.40**	**12.94**	**9.99**	**2.51**	**40.32**	**0.016**
Praying/Hope	21.80	6.14	22.58	8.64	−0.35	37.58	0.727
Declaring coping	21.27	5.87	19.13	8.93	0.97	39.68	0.339
Increased behavioral activity	20.80	6.35	19.13	9.54	0.70	39.37	0.485

M.- average value; SD - standard deviation; t - value of the Student's t-test; df - the number of degrees of freedom; p - statistical significance.

Table 10.
Average values of the strategies of coping with pain in the group of people who were treated with radiotherapy and in the group of people who were not treated with radiotherapy.

Targeted treatment							
	Yes		no				
Variable	*M.*	*SD*	*M.*	*SD*	*vol*	*df*	*p*
Distraction	19.50	4.30	19.19	8.81	0.15	31.27	0.880
Re-evaluation of pain sensations	**19.00**	**4.40**	**11.78**	**9.65**	**3.40**	**33.69**	**0.002**
Catastrophizing	20.30	4.27	17.86	8.32	0.89	44	0.378
Ignoring sensations	**21.60**	**4.09**	**13.08**	**9.60**	**4.14**	**35.99**	**0.001**
Praying/Hope	21.60	6.10	22.53	8.34	−0.33	44	0.745
Declaring coping	24.20	6.76	18.61	8.05	2.00	44	0.051
Increased behavioral activity	21.70	3.43	19.11	9.51	1.35	40.70	0.185

M.- average value; SD - standard deviation; t - value of the Student's t-test; df - the number of degrees of freedom; p - statistical significance.

Table 11.
Mean values of the strategies of coping with pain in the group of people who were undergoing targeted therapy and in the group of people who were not undergoing targeted therapy.

It was found that the mean values of the fighting spirit and positive re-evaluation were statistically significantly higher than the mean value of the helplessness-hopelessness index.

Table 12 presents the mean values of the mental adjustment indices in the group of women and in the group of men. The list was supplemented with the values of the Student's two-sided t-test for independent samples.

There was a statistically significant difference in terms of the positive re-evaluation strategy.

Table 13 shows the Pearson r correlation coefficients between the age of the respondents and the psychological adjustment indices. Statistically significant correlations were marked.

Statistically significant positive correlations were obtained between the age of the respondents and the fighting spirit index and a positive re-evaluation.

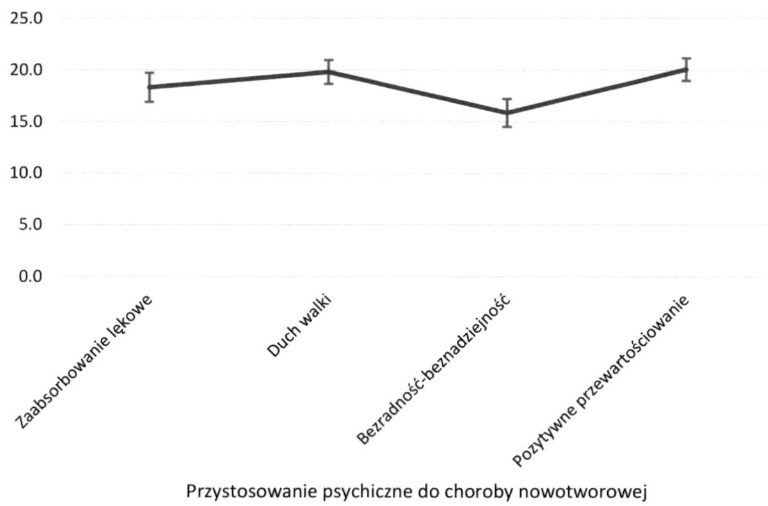

Figure 4.
The mean values of the indicators of mental adaptation to neoplastic disease with confidence intervals determined based on the Bonferroni correction.

	Women		Men				
Variable	*M.*	*SD*	*M.*	*SD*	*vol*	*df*	*p*
Anxiety preoccupation	18.88	3.72	17.68	5.64	0.84	35.88	0.407
Fighting spirit	19.96	4.53	19.64	3.13	0.28	44	0.782
Helplessness-hopelessness	16.08	3.89	15.64	5.28	0.33	44	0.744
Positive reevaluation	**21.63**	**3.05**	**18.36**	**3.58**	**3.34**	**44**	**0.002**

M.- average value; SD - standard deviation; t - value of the Student's t-test; df - the number of degrees of freedom; p - statistical significance.

Table 12.
Average values of mental adjustment indicators in the group of women and in the group of men.

Variables	Age
Anxiety preoccupation	−0.022
Fighting spirit	0.429*
Helplessness-hopelessness	−0.195
Positive reevaluation	0.550*

$^*p < 0.01$.

Table 13.
Pearson's r correlation coefficients between the age of the respondents and the indicators of mental adjustment.

Table 14 shows the average values of the adaptation rates in the group of people with primary or vocational education, in the group of people with secondary education and in the group of people with higher education. The summary was supplemented with the values of one-way analysis of variance.

Statistically significant differences were obtained in terms of a positive re-evaluation. On the basis of Gabriel's post-hoc test, it was found that statistically significant differences existed between people with higher education and people

	Education							
	basic/valve		medium		higher			
Variable	*M.*	*SD*	*M.*	*SD*	*M.*	*SD*	*F.*	*p*
Anxiety preoccupation	18.31	4.39	18.71	5.50	17.94	4.60	0.10	0.908
Fighting spirit	21.50	3.33	18.86	4.88	18.94	2.98	2.49	0.095
Helplessness-hopelessness	15.50	4.75	15.71	5.04	16.38	4.16	0.15	0.859
Positive reevaluation	21.00	2.58	21.93	3.20	17.50	3.69	8.26	0.001

M.- average value; SD - standard deviation; F - value of the one-way analysis of variance; p - statistical significance.

Table 14.
Average values of the adaptation indicators in the group of people with primary or vocational education, in the group of people with secondary education and in the group of people with higher education.

with primary or vocational education, $p < 0.05$, and people with secondary education, $p < 0.01$.

Table 15 shows the average values of the adaptation indicators in the group of people living in towns with a population of up to 100,000 and in the group of people living in towns with more than 100,000 inhabitants. The list was supplemented with the values of Student's two-sided t-test for independent samples.

There were no statistically significant differences.

Table 16 shows the average values of the adaptation rates in the group of people with an average monthly net income per family member of up to PLN 1,500 and in the group of people with an average monthly net income per family member above PLN 1,500. The list was supplemented with the values of Student's two-sided t-test for independent samples.

A statistically significant difference was obtained in terms of a positive re-evaluation.

Table 17 shows the average values of the adaptation indicators in the group of working people and in the group of retirees and pensioners. The list was supplemented with the values of Student's two-sided t-test for independent samples.

A statistically significant difference was obtained in terms of a positive re-evaluation.

	The number of residents						
	up to 100,000		over 100 thousand				
Variable	*M.*	*SD*	*M.*	*SD*	*vol*	*df*	*p*
Anxiety preoccupation	17.81	4.70	18.95	4.80	−0.81	44	0.422
Fighting spirit	19.96	3.75	19.60	4.15	0.31	44	0.758
Helplessness-hopelessness	14.81	4.20	17.25	4.74	−1.85	44	0.071
Positive reevaluation	20.81	3.07	19.10	4.20	1.59	44	0.118

M.- average value; SD - standard deviation; t - value of the Student's t-test; df - the number of degrees of freedom; p - statistical significance.

Table 15.
Average values of adaptation indicators in the group of people living in towns with a population of up to 100,000 and in the group of people living in towns with more than 100,000 inhabitants.

	Average monthly net income						
	up to PLN 1,500		**over 1500 zlotys**				
Variable	*M.*	*SD*	*M.*	*SD*	*vol*	*df*	*p*
Anxiety preoccupation	17.70	4.77	18.91	4.70	−0.87	44	0.388
Fighting spirit	20.13	3.42	19.48	4.36	0.56	44	0.575
Helplessness-hopelessness	15.17	4.75	16.57	4.35	−1.04	44	0.306
Positive reevaluation	**21.57**	**2.52**	**18.57**	**4.05**	**3.01**	**44**	**0.004**

M.- average value; SD - standard deviation; t - value of the Student's t-test; df - the number of degrees of freedom; p - statistical significance.

Table 16.
Average values of adaptation indicators in the group of people with an average monthly net income per family member up to PLN 1,500 and in the group of people with an average monthly net income per family member above PLN 1,500.

	Professional status						
	working		**retirees/pensioners**				
Variable	*M.*	*SD*	*M.*	*SD*	*vol*	*df*	*p*
Anxiety preoccupation	17.95	5.17	18.57	4.67	−0.41	41	0.684
Fighting spirit	19.30	2.79	20.65	4.65	−1.13	41	0.263
Helplessness-hopelessness	16.45	4.84	15.39	4.42	0.75	41	0.458
Positive reevaluation	**17.70**	**3.69**	**21.83**	**2.52**	**−4.33**	**41**	**0.001**

M.- average value; SD - standard deviation; t - value of the Student's t-test; df - the number of degrees of freedom; p - statistical significance.

Table 17.
Average values of adaptation indicators in the group of working people and in the group of retirees and disability pensioners.

Table 18 presents the mean values of the adaptation indices in the group of people with diagnosed metastases and in the group of people with no diagnosis of metastases. The list was supplemented with the values of Student's two-sided t-test for independent samples.

A statistically significant difference was obtained in terms of the fighting spirit index.

	Known metastases						
	Yes		**no**				
Variable	*M.*	*SD*	*M.*	*SD*	*vol*	*df*	*p*
Anxiety preoccupation	18.52	4.10	17.67	5.14	0.61	42	0.543
Fighting spirit	**18.70**	**3.85**	**21.10**	**3.58**	**−2.13**	**42**	**0.039**
Helplessness-hopelessness	16.57	3.95	14.76	4.71	1.38	42	0.175
Positive reevaluation	19.39	3.30	21.33	3.51	−1.89	42	0.066

M.- average value; SD - standard deviation; t - value of the Student's t-test; df - the number of degrees of freedom; p - statistical significance.

Table 18.
Average values of the adaptation indices in the group of people with diagnosed metastases and in the group of people without metastases.

Table 19 shows the mean values of the adaptation indices in the group of people who were undergoing chemotherapeutic treatment and in the group of people who were not undergoing chemotherapy. The list was supplemented with the values of Student's two-sided t-test for independent samples.

No statistically significant differences were found.

Table 20 shows the mean values of the adaptation indices in the group of people who were undergoing chemotherapy treatment and in the group of people who were not undergoing chemotherapy. The list was supplemented with the values of Student's two-sided t-test for independent samples.

There were no statistically significant differences.

Table 21 presents the mean values of the adaptation indices in the group of people who were treated with radiotherapy and in the group of people who were not treated with radiotherapy. The list was supplemented with the values of Student's two-sided t-test for independent samples.

A statistically significant difference was obtained in terms of a positive reevaluation.

Table 22 presents the mean values of the adaptation indices in the group of people who were under targeted treatment and in the group of people who were not under targeted therapy. The list was supplemented with the values of Student's two-sided t-test for independent samples.

No statistically significant intergroup differences were obtained.

	Chemotherapeutic treatment						
	Yes		**no**				
Variable	*M.*	*SD*	*M.*	*SD*	*vol*	*df*	*p*
Anxiety preoccupation	18.44	4.62	18.14	4.95	0.21	44	0.834
Fighting spirit	18.96	3.22	20.81	4.42	−1.64	44	0.109
Helplessness-hopelessness	16.44	4.41	15.19	4.75	0.92	44	0.360
Positive reevaluation	19.16	3.25	21.14	3.92	−1.88	44	0.067

M.- average value; SD - standard deviation; t - value of the Student's t-test; df - the number of degrees of freedom; p - statistical significance.

Table 19.
Average values of adaptation indices in the group of people who were undergoing chemotherapy treatment and in the group of people who were not undergoing chemotherapeutic treatment.

	Chemotherapeutic treatment						
	Yes		**no**				
Variable	*M.*	*SD*	*M.*	*SD*	*vol*	*df*	*p*
Anxiety preoccupation	18.44	4.62	18.14	4.95	0.21	44	0.834
Fighting spirit	18.96	3.22	20.81	4.42	−1.64	44	0.109
Helplessness-hopelessness	16.44	4.41	15.19	4.75	0.92	44	0.360
Positive reevaluation	19.16	3.25	21.14	3.92	−1.88	44	0.067

M.- average value; SD - standard deviation; t - value of the Student's t-test; df - the number of degrees of freedom; p - statistical significance.

Table 20.
Average values of adaptation indices in the group of people who were undergoing chemotherapy treatment and in the group of people who were not undergoing chemotherapeutic treatment.

	Treatment with radiation therapy						
	Yes		no				
Variable	*M.*	*SD*	*M.*	*SD*	*vol*	*df*	*p*
Anxiety preoccupation	17.73	4.62	18.58	4.82	−0.57	44	0.574
Fighting spirit	18.80	4.31	20.29	3.63	−1.23	44	0.227
Helplessness-hopelessness	15.33	3.68	16.13	4.96	−0.61	36.38	0.545
Positive reevaluation	**18.53**	**4.07**	**20.81**	**3.27**	**−2.04**	**44**	**0.047**

M.- average value; SD - standard deviation; t - value of the Student's t-test; df - the number of degrees of freedom; p - statistical significance.

Table 21.
Average values of adaptation indicators in the group of people who were treated with radiotherapy and in the group of people who were not treated with radiotherapy.

	Targeted treatment						
	Yes		no				
Variable	*M.*	*SD*	*M.*	*SD*	*vol*	*df*	*p*
Anxiety preoccupation	18.00	3.16	18.39	5.11	−0.23	44	0.821
Fighting spirit	19.60	3.37	19.86	4.06	−0.19	44	0.853
Helplessness-hopelessness	17.20	2.66	15.50	4.93	1.45	27.84	0.159
Positive reevaluation	18.10	3.31	20.61	3.61	−1.98	44	0.054

M.- average value; SD - standard deviation; t - value of the Student's t-test; df - the number of degrees of freedom; p - statistical significance.

Table 22.
Average values of adaptation indices in the group of people who were under targeted treatment and in the group of people who were not under targeted treatment.

A.1.4 Acceptance of the disease

The mean value of disease acceptance in the group of women was 22.54 with the standard deviation of 7.39, which was close to the mean value in the group of men, which was 23.77 with the standard deviation of 8.43. Based on the value of the Student's t-test for independent samples, it was found that the difference obtained was statistically insignificant, t (44) = − 0.53, p > 0.05.

The disease acceptance did not correlate statistically with the age of the patients, r (44) = 0.03, p > 0.05.

The mean value of disease acceptance in the group of people with primary or vocational education was 22.08 with the standard deviation equal to 8.07, in the group with secondary education it was 23.43 with the standard deviation equal to 10.00, and in the group with higher education it was 23, 13 with a standard deviation of 5.69. Based on the value of the one-way analysis of variance, it was found that the obtained differences were statistically insignificant, F (2.43) = 0.02, p > 0.05.

The mean value of disease acceptance in the group of people living in towns with a population of up to 100,000 was 23.12 with a standard deviation of 7.45 and was close to the average value obtained in the group of people who lived in towns with more than 100,000 inhabitants, 23, 15 with a standard deviation of 8.51. Based on the value of the Student's t-test for independent samples, it was found that the obtained difference was statistically insignificant, t (44) = − 0.01, p > 0.05.

The mean value of disease acceptance in the group of people with a net income of up to PLN 1,500 was 23.61 with a standard deviation of 8.65 and was close to the average value obtained in the group of people with income above PLN 1,500, which was 22.65 with a standard deviation of 7, 09. Based on the value of the Student's t-test for independent samples, it was found that the obtained difference was statistically insignificant, $t(44) = -0.41$, $p > 0.05$.

The mean value of disease acceptance in the working group was 24.85 with a standard deviation of 7.05 and was close to the mean value in the group of retirees and disability pensioners of 21.52 with a standard deviation of 8.70. Based on the value of the Student's t-test for independent samples, it was found that the obtained difference was statistically insignificant, $t(41) = 1.37$, $p > 0.05$.

The mean value of disease acceptance in the group of people diagnosed with metastases was 21.70 with a standard deviation of 6.00 and was close to the mean value of 25.05 in the group of non-metastatic patients with a standard deviation of 8.83. Based on the value of the Student's t-test for independent samples, it was found that the obtained difference was statistically insignificant, $t(34.78) = -1.46$, $p > 0.05$.

The mean disease acceptance value in the group of people who were on chemotherapy treatment was 22.84 with a standard deviation of 7.98, which was close to the mean value for the group of people who were not on chemotherapy treatment of 23.48 with a standard deviation of 7, 85. Based on the value of the Student's t-test for independent samples, it was found that the obtained difference was statistically insignificant, $t(44) = -0.27$, $p > 0.05$.

The mean disease acceptance value in the group of people who received radiotherapy was 24.87 with a standard deviation of 5.68 and was close to the mean value in the group of people who did not receive radiotherapy was 22.29 with a standard deviation of 8, 65. Based on the value of the Student's t-test for independent samples, it was found that the obtained difference was not statistically significant, $t(39.27) = 1.21$, $p > 0.05$.

The mean disease acceptance value in the group of people who were on targeted treatment was 25.70 with a standard deviation of 3.86 and was close to the mean value in the group of people who did not receive targeted therapy was 22.42 with a standard deviation of 8, 53. Based on the value of the Student's t-test for independent samples, it was found that the obtained difference was statistically insignificant, $t(33.93) = 1.75$, $p > 0.05$.

A.1.5 Pain control

Table 23 shows the mean values of pain control dimensions in the men and women groups. The list was supplemented with the values of Student's two-sided t-test for independent samples.

There was a statistically significant difference in the internal locus of pain control.

Table 24 shows the Pearson r correlation coefficients between the age of the subjects and the dimensions of pain control.

No statistically significant correlations were obtained.

Table 25 shows the mean values of pain control dimensions in the group of people with primary or vocational education, in the group of people with secondary education, and in the group of people with higher education. The summary was supplemented with the values of one-way analysis of variance.

No statistically significant differences were obtained.

Table 26 shows the mean values of pain control dimensions in the group of people living in towns with a population of up to 100,000 and in the group of people living in towns with more than 100,000 inhabitants. The list was supplemented with the values of Student's two-sided t-test for independent samples.

	Women		Men				
Variable	*M.*	*SD*	*M.*	*SD*	*vol*	*df*	*p*
Inside	**18.63**	**6.29**	**14.91**	**4.15**	**2.34**	**44**	**0.024**
The influence of doctors	17.21	3.82	15.82	4.57	1.12	44	0.268
Random events	15.63	4.25	14.00	3.87	1.35	44	0.183

M.- average value; SD - standard deviation; t - value of the Student's t-test; df - the number of degrees of freedom; p - statistical significance.

Table 23.
Mean values of pain control dimensions in the group of women and the group of men.

The site of pain control	Age
Inside	−0.009
The influence of doctors	−0.022
Random events	0.186

Table 24.
Pearson's r correlation coefficients between the age of the subjects and the dimensions of pain control.

	Education							
	basic/valve		medium		higher			
Variable	*M.*	*SD*	*M.*	*SD*	*M.*	*SD*	*F.*	*p*
Inside	16.13	5.49	17.71	6.65	16.81	5.06	0.29	0.751
The influence of doctors	14.81	5.47	17.57	3.39	17.38	2.90	2.19	0.124
Random events	14.63	4.51	14.36	4.48	15.50	3.48	0.31	0.732

M.- average value; SD - standard deviation; F - value of the one-way analysis of variance; p - statistical significance.

Table 25.
Mean values of pain control dimensions in the group of people with primary or vocational education, in the group of people with secondary education and in the group of people with higher education.

	The number of residents						
	up to 100,000		over 100 thousand				
Variable	*M.*	*SD*	*M.*	*SD*	*vol*	*df*	*p*
Inside	17.15	5.45	16.45	6.00	0.42	44	0.679
The influence of doctors	16.27	4.61	16.90	3.71	−0.50	44	0.620
Random events	15.19	4.68	14.40	3.28	0.64	44	0.523

M.- average value; SD - standard deviation; t - value of the Student's t-test; df - the number of degrees of freedom; p - statistical significance.

Table 26.
Average values of pain control dimensions in the group of people living in towns with a population of up to 100,000 and in the group of people living in towns with more than 100,000 inhabitants.

There were no statistically significant differences.

Table 27 shows the mean values of pain control dimensions in the group of people with an average monthly net income per family member of up to PLN 1,500 and in the group of people with an average monthly net income per family member

	Average monthly net income						
	up to PLN 1,500		**over 1500 zlotys**				
Variable	*M.*	*SD*	*M.*	*SD*	*vol*	*df*	*p*
Inside	16.43	5.86	17.26	5.50	−0.49	44	0.625
The influence of doctors	16.30	4.12	16.78	4.38	−0.38	44	0.705
Random events	**13.52**	**4.08**	**16.17**	**3.77**	**−2.29**	**44**	**0.027**

M.- average value; SD - standard deviation; t - value of the Student's t-test; df - the number of degrees of freedom; p - statistical significance.

Table 27.
Average values of pain control dimensions in the group of people with an average monthly net income per family member up to PLN 1,500 and in the group of people with an average monthly net income per family member above PLN 1,500.

above PLN 1,500. The list was supplemented with the values of Student's two-sided t-test for independent samples.

A statistically significant difference was found in the location of pain control in random events.

Table 28 shows the mean values of pain control dimensions in the working group and in the group of retirees and pensioners. The list was supplemented with the values of Student's two-sided t-test for independent samples.

No statistically significant differences were obtained.

Table 29 shows the mean values of the dimensions of pain control in the group of patients with diagnosed metastases and in the group of individuals without diagnosis. The list was supplemented with the values of Student's two-sided t-test for independent samples.

	Professional status						
	working		**retirees/pensioners**				
Variable	*M.*	*SD*	*M.*	*SD*	*vol*	*df*	*p*
Inside	15.95	4.47	17.04	6.58	−0.63	41	0.534
The influence of doctors	16.65	3.59	16.61	4.93	0.03	41	0.975
Random events	14.30	3.76	15.39	4.44	−0.86	41	0.393

M.- average value; SD - standard deviation; t - value of the Student's t-test; df - the number of degrees of freedom; p - statistical significance.

Table 28.
Mean values of pain control dimensions in the working group and in the group of retirees and pensioners.

	Known metastases						
	Yes		**no**				
Variable	*M.*	*SD*	*M.*	*SD*	*vol*	*df*	*p*
Inside	16.39	5.19	17.38	5.84	−0.60	42	0.555
The influence of doctors	16.52	4.28	16.14	4.17	0.30	42	0.768
Random events	14.87	3.51	14.90	4.85	−0.03	42	0.978

M.- average value; SD - standard deviation; t - value of the Student's t-test; df - the number of degrees of freedom; p - statistical significance.

Table 29.
Mean values of pain control dimensions in the group of people who have not been diagnosed with metastases.

No statistically significant differences were obtained.

Table 30 shows the mean values of the dimensions of pain control in the group of subjects who received chemotherapy and the group of subjects who were not receiving chemotherapy. The list was supplemented with the values of Student's two-sided t-test for independent samples.

No statistically significant differences were obtained.

Table 31 shows the mean values of the dimensions of pain control in the group of people who were treated with radiotherapy and in the group who were not

	Chemotherapeutic treatment						
	Yes		no				
Variable	*M.*	*SD*	*M.*	*SD*	*vol*	*df*	*p*
Inside	17.24	4.85	16.38	6.55	0.51	44	0.612
The influence of doctors	15.92	4.21	17.29	4.19	−1.10	44	0.278
Random events	13.80	2.50	16.10	5.24	−1.84	27.532	0.077

M.- average value; SD - standard deviation, t - value of the Student's t-test; df - the number of degrees of freedom; p statistical significance.

Table 30.
Mean values of pain control dimensions in the group of people who were undergoing chemotherapy treatment and in the group of people who were not undergoing chemotherapy treatment.

	Treatment with radiation therapy						
	Yes		no				
Variable	*M.*	*SD*	*M.*	*SD*	*vol*	*df*	*p*
Inside	16.53	3.78	17.00	6.40	−0.26	44	0.796
The influence of doctors	**14.60**	**3.36**	**17.48**	**4.30**	**−2.28**	**44**	**0.028**
Random events	14.20	2.76	15.16	4.63	−0.88	41.90	0.385

M.- average value; SD - standard deviation; t - value of the Student's t-test; df - the number of degrees of freedom; p - statistical significance.

Table 31.
Mean values of the dimensions of pain control in the group of people who were treated with radiotherapy and in the group of people who were not treated with radiotherapy.

	Targeted treatment						
	Yes		no				
Variable	*M.*	*SD*	*M.*	*SD*	*vol*	*df*	*p*
Inside	16.80	4.44	16.86	5.98	−0.03	44	0.976
The influence of doctors	15.00	2.36	16.97	4.53	−1.86	29.04	0.073
Random events	14.60	3.81	14.92	4.24	−0.21	44	0.832

M.- average value; SD - standard deviation; t - value of the Student's t-test; df - the number of degrees of freedom; p - statistical significance.

Table 32.
Mean values of pain control dimensions in the group of people who were undergoing targeted treatment and in the group of people who were not undergoing targeted therapy.

treated with radiation therapy. The list was supplemented with the values of Student's two-sided t-test for independent samples.

A statistically significant intergroup difference was obtained in the location of pain control in the influence of doctors.

Table 32 shows the mean values of the dimensions of pain control in the group of people who were on targeted therapy and in the group of people who were not on targeted therapy. The list was supplemented with the values of Student's two-sided t-test for independent samples.

No statistically significant differences were obtained.

Author details

Urszula Religioni[1*], Aleksandra Czerw[2,3], Anna M. Badowska-Kozakiewicz[4], Michał Budzik[4] and Andrzej Deptała[4,5]

1 Collegium of Business Administration, Warsaw School of Economics, Warsaw, Poland

2 Department of Health Economics and Medical Law, Medical University of Warsaw, Warsaw, Poland

3 Department of Economic and System Analyses, National Institute of Public Health - NIH, Warsaw, Poland

4 Department of Cancer Prevention, Medical University of Warsaw, Warsaw, Poland

5 Department of Oncology and Hematology, Central Clinical Hospital of the MSWiA in Warsaw, Warsaw, Poland

*Address all correspondence to: urszula.religioni@gmail.com

References

[1] Wojciechowska U, Czaderny K, Ciuba A, Olasek P, Didkowska J. Cancer in Poland in 2016. National Cancer Registry 2016. http://onkologia.org.pl/wp-content/uploads/Nowotwory_2016.pdf, 05.07.2017. Accessed 16 September 2019.

[2] Ilic M, Ilic I. Epidemiology of pancreatic cancer. *World J Gastroenterol* 2016; 22(44): 9694–9705.

[3] Siegel RL, Miller KD, Jemal A. Cancer Statistics. *CA Cancer J Clin* 2019; 69:7–34.

[4] Zhang Q, Zeng L, Chen Y et al. Pancreatic Cancer Epidemiology, Detection, and Management. *Gastroenterol Res Pract* 2016: 8962321.

[5] Malafa MP, Al-Hawary M, Asbun H et al. Pancreatic adenocarcinoma, version 2.2017: NCCN Clinical Practice Guidelines in Oncology. *J Natl Compr Canc Netw* 2017; 15(8): 1028-1061.

[6] Gooden HM, White KJ. Pancreatic cancer and supportive care—pancreatic exocrine insufficiency negatively impacts on quality of life. *Supportive Care in Cancer* 2013; 21(7): 1835–1841.

[7] Carrato A, Falcone A, Ducreux M et al. A Systematic Review of the Burden of Pancreatic Cancer in Europe: Real-World Impact on Survival, Quality of Life and Costs. *J Gastrointest Canc* 2015; 46(3): 201-211.

[8] Skevington SM. A standardized scale to measure beliefs about controlling pain (BPCQ): a preliminary study. *Psychol Health* 1990; 4: 221-232.

[9] Rosenstiel AK, Keefe FJ. The use of cognitive doping strategies in chronic low back pain patients: relationship to patient characteristics and current adjustment. *Pain* 1983; 17: 33-44.

[10] Felton BJ, Revenson TA, Hinrichsen GA. Stress and coping in the explanation of psychological adjustment among chronically ill adults. *Soc Sci Med* 1984; 18(10): 889–898.

[11] Watson M, Law M, Santos M, Greer S, Baruch J, Bliss J. The Mini-MAC: further development of the Mental Adjustment to Cancer Scale. *J Psych Oncol* 1994; 12(3): 33-46.

[12] Krupas D, Kusz J, Jedynak T, Mroczek B. The acceptance level of chronic diseases among patients. *Family Med Prim Care Rev* 2012; 14(3): 396–398.

[13] Zylicz Z. Palliative care for the patients with pancreatic cancer. *Medycyna Paliatywna w Praktyce* 2014; 8 (4): 145–151.

[14] Zielińska D, Durlik M. Quality of life in patients after pancreas resection – review paper. *Prz Gastroenterol* 2010; 5 (2): 83–87.

[15] Zabora J, Brintzenhofe-Szoc K, Curbow B, Hooker C, Piantadosi S. The prevalence of psychological distress by cancer site. *Psycho-oncology* 2001; 10(1): 19-28.

[16] Clark KL, Loscalzo M, Trask PC, Zabora J, Philip EJ. Psychological distress in patients with pancreatic cancer - an understudied group. *Psycho-oncology* 2010; 19(12): 1313-1320.

[17] Basińska MA, Andruszkiewicz A. Locus of pain control and coping strategies with chronic pain by patients treated for lung cancer and colorectal cancer. *Psychoonkologia* 2014; 2: 43–50.

[18] Suchocka L. Psychologia bólu. Difin Publishing House.Warsaw, 2008.

[19] Masters KS, Wallston KA. Canonical correlation reveals important relations

between health locus of control, coping, affect and values. *J Health Psychol* 2005; 10: 719-731.

[20] Czerw A, Religioni U, Deptała A, Walewska-Zielecka B. Assessment of pain, acceptance of illness, adjustment to life with cancer, and coping strategies in colorectal cancer patients. *Prz Gastroenterol* 2016; 11(2): 96–103.

[21] Czerw A, Religioni U, Deptała A, Fronczak A. Pain, acceptance of illness, adjustment to life with cancer and coping strategies in prostate cancer patients. *Arch Med Sci* 2017; 13(6): 1459–1466.

[22] Czerw A, Religioni U, Deptała A. Adjustment to Life with Lung Cancer. *Adv Clin Exp Med* 2016; 25(4): 733–740.

[23] Czerw A, Religioni U, Deptała A. Assessment of pain, acceptance of illness, adjustment to life with cancer and coping strategies in breast cancer patients. *Breast Cancer* 2016; 23(4): 654–661.

[24] Religioni U, Czerw A, Deptała A. Strategies of Coping with Pain in Cancer on the Basis of Lung, Breast, Colorectal, and Prostate Carcinoma. *J Canc Edu* 2017; 32(4): 771-777.

[25] McCracken L, Eccleston C. A comparison of the relative of coping and acceptance-based measures in a sample of chronic pain sufferers. *Eur J Pain* 2006; 10:23-29.

[26] Merlijn VP, Hunfeld JA, van der Wonden JC. Factors related to the quality of life in adolescents with chronic pain. *Clin J Pain* 2006; 22: 306-315.

[27] Religioni U, Czerw A, Deptała A. Acceptance of Cancer in Patients Diagnosed with Lung, Breast, Colorectal and Prostate Carcinoma. *Iran J Public Health* 2015; 44(8): 1135–1142.

[28] Kapela I, Bąk E, Krzemińska SA, Fołtyn A. Evaluation of the level of acceptance of the disease and of satisfaction with life in patients with colorectal cancer treated with chemotherapy. *Nursing and Public Health* 2017; 26(1): 53–61.

[29] Kozak G. Different strategies of managing neoplasia in the course of chosen cancers. *Anestezjologia i Ratownictwo* 2012; 6: 162-170.

[30] Kołpa M, Wywrot-Kozłowska B, Jurkiewicz B, Grochowska A. The factors determining acceptance and adjustment to cancer. *Pielęgniarstwo Chirurgiczne i Angiologiczne* 2015; 3: 165–169.

[31] Juczyński Z. Assessment tools in health promotion and psychology. Laboratory of Psychological Tests of the Polish Psychological Association, Warsaw, 2001.

[32] Bussel V, Naus M. A longitudinal investigation of coping and posttraumatic growth in breast cancer survivors. *J Psychosoc Oncol* 2010; 28: 61-78.

[33] Religioni U, Czerw A, Deptała A. Patient mental adjustment to selected types of cancer. *Psychiatr Pol* 2018; 52 (1): 129–141.

[34] Augustynowicz A, Czerw A, Deptała A. Health needs as a priority of local authorities in Poland based on the example of implementation of health policy cancer programmes. *Arch Med Sci* 2018; 14(6): 1439–1449.

[35] Juczyński Z. Coping with stress caused by cancer). [in:] De Walden Gałuszko K (ed.). Psychoonkologia. Publishing House of the Polish Psychiatric Association, Kraków: 23-43, 2000.

[36] Bahnson C, Bahnson M, Wardwell W. A psychological study of cancer: Abstracts. *Psychosomatic Medicine* 1991; 5:53-85.

Chapter 4

Predictors of Health-Related Quality of Life among Patients with Diabetes Mellitus

Bikila Regassa Feyisa

Abstract

The health of general population cannot be well characterized from the analyses of mortality and morbidity statistics alone, particularly for patients of chronic diseases including diabetes mellitus. It is equally important to contemplate health in terms of people's assessment of their sense of well-being and ability to perform social roles. A number of reasons are there to measure the health-related quality of life among patients with diabetes mellitus. For one thing, diabetes patients are highly interested in functional capacity and well-being. On the other hand, patients in the same clinical manifestations might have different responses. Either general or specific instruments could be utilized to measure the health-related quality of life of diabetes patients. Choice of the instrument depends on time of the measurement, validity of the instrument and the interpretability. In Ethiopia, short form 36 (SF-36) instruments were utilized and the highest (63.2 $\pm$ 34.4) and the lowest (30.2 $\pm$ 22.9) mean score scored in physical functioning and general health domain respectively. The study indicated that age, sex, marital status, educational status, feeling of stigmatized, co-morbidity status, chronic complication and body mass index are some of the predictors of health-related quality of life for patients living with diabetes mellitus.

Keywords: Health-related quality of life, diabetes mellitus, Ethiopia

1. Introduction

Diabetes mellitus (DM) is a chronic disease that occurs when the pancreas fails to produce enough insulin or when the body's insulin is not used correctly. There are numerous forms of diabetes, and each form is caused by a complex mix of genetics and environmental factors. Type 1 and type 2 diabetes mellitus are two basic classifications of the disease. Chronic high blood glucose levels (>126 mg/dl for fasting blood sugar and/or a 2-hour postprandial glucose of 200 mg/dl, or if the individual experienced symptoms of diabetes and random plasma glucose of 200 mg/dl (confirmed by repeat testing) are indications of diabetes [1–3].

Diabetes mellitus (DM) is a rising condition that has a significant influence on health and quality of life. It is seen as a pressing public health issue that has the potential to negatively impact health-related quality of life [2, 4, 5]. In 2015, around 8.8% of persons aged 20 to 79 had diabetes worldwide. Over 2030, this tendency is expected to reach 366 million cases, rising to 642 million cases (one in every ten individuals) by the next decade. Around 75% of them were from low- and

IntechOpen

middle-income nations. Diabetes was responsible for over 5 million deaths worldwide between the ages of 20 and 99 [6–8].

The increasing burden of diabetes has also great economic impact directly for medical costs and indirectly by loss of jobs and wages. The global healthcare expenditure on people with diabetes was estimated to be USD 850 billion in 2017 [3, 8].

There is now an universal agreement that the general population's health cannot be adequately assessed solely through the analysis of mortality and morbidity statistics, and that health must also be considered in terms of people's perceptions of their sense of well-being and ability to perform social roles [9, 10].

This evaluation could be correct if the health-related quality of life of individuals, particularly those with chronic illness, could be accurately assessed. The phrase "health-related quality of life" (HRQoL) refers to a multifaceted notion that considers how patients are affected by sickness and treatment. It can assess patients' views of sickness and treatment, as well as their perceived needs for healthcare providers, treatment preferences, and disease outcomes [11, 12].

The subjective and objective assessments of an individual with particular conditions are included in health-related quality of life. The word is used because there are many parts of life that are highly valued but are not considered to be "healthy." It's been described as "an overall general well-being that includes objective descriptors and subjective evaluations of physical, material, social, and emotional well-being, as well as the extent of personal development and purposeful activity, all weighted by a personal set of values [13]."

Although clinicians and experienced professionals can assess the severity of the condition and the extent to which it has progressed, their assessment of the clients' health-related quality of life may differ from the patients' personal perspective. This is because psychosocial and cultural factors may have a significant impact on patients' personal perspectives [3].

Diabetes mellitus has a negative impact on patients' HRQoL. This, in turn, has an impact on many aspects of a person's life, including the psychological impact of being chronically ill, dietary restrictions, social changes, and imprecise symptoms of an inadequate metabolic system, chronic complications, and, eventually, lifelong infirmities [14, 15].

The objective of chronic care are not to cure but to enhance functional status, minimize distressing symptoms, prolong life through secondary prevention and improve the quality of life [16].

Diabetes Mellitus also has a profound effect on social, economic, physical, psychological, behavioral and clinical conditions of the person affected. These effects will have a great impact on the health-related quality of life and it is one of the most psychologically demanding of the chronic diseases; with psychosocial factors pertinent to nearly every aspect of the disease and its treatment [11].

2. Health-related quality of life and chronic diseases

Health status, functional status, and quality of life are the three categories of health that are most frequently used interchangeably [17]. The health domains vary from death, which is one of life's adversely valued features, to extreme happiness or full functioning, which is one of life's favorably valued aspects. The rationale for assessing health and the specific concerns of patients, clinicians, and researchers in the subject of study usually determine the definition's boundaries.

While income level, independence, and environmental quality may all play a role in determining HRQoL, they do not directly affect people's health or medical concerns. HRQoL is the right focus for clinicians, having in mind that when a patient is suffering from disease or illness, practically every area of their life might become health-related.

3. Why measure health-related quality of life?

Measuring HRQoL is becoming more widely accepted as a means of assessing the effects of chronic illness [18]. Physiological measurements are useful for physicians, but they are of little interest to patients, and they often have poor correlations with functional capability and well-being, which are the areas in which patients are most interested. Variations in exercise capacity among patients evaluated in the laboratory, for example, are very weakly connected to differences in the ability to conduct day-to-day activities in patients with chronic heart and lung illness [19]. Another reason to test HRQoL is the typical occurrence of two patients with the same clinical criteria having vastly different responses. Two patients with the same forced expiratory volume in 1 s and even the same exercise capacity in the lab, for example, may have different role functions and emotional well-being. While one patient may be able to continue working without experiencing sadness, another may be forced to leave their job and suffer from a major depression [19, 20].

These reasons explain why the impact of medical therapies on HRQoL are of great interest to patients, doctors, and healthcare executives [20]. HRQoL is of special importance to managers since the patient mix influences consumption and expenditure patterns. HRQoL is increasingly being used as a measure of care quality and clinical efficacy, and payers are beginning to factor HRQoL data into payment decisions.

4. Types of health-related quality of life measures

4.1 Generic instruments-health profile

HRQoL assessments can be classified into two categories: generic and specific. Single indicators, health profiles, and utility measures are some of the generic instruments available. Health profiles are tools that seek to quantify all components of HRQoL. The Sickness Impact Profile (SIP) is a health profile that includes a physical dimension (ambulation, mobility, body care, and movement); a psychosocial dimension (social interaction, alertness behavior, communication, and emotional behavior); and five independent categories (eating, work, home management, sleep and rest, recreations, and pastimes). Because of its broad breadth, using health profiles provides an advantage. Generic instruments allow for comprehensive evaluations of the relative impact of various healthcare initiatives since they apply to a wide variety of people. Generic profiles, on the other hand, may be less responsive to changes in specific situations [21].

4.2 Specific instruments

The second basic strategy to assessing quality of life focuses on features of health that are relevant to the major concern. The reason for this strategy is that it has the potential to boost responsiveness by focusing on only the most significant parts of HRQoL that is relevant to the patients being examined. The instrument could be tailored to a condition (such as diabetes or heart failure), a patient demographic (such as the frail elderly), a specific function (such as sleep or sexual function), or a problem (such as pain). Aside from the possibility of better responsiveness, specific measures have the advantage of being directly related to areas that clinicians usually investigate.

Health-related quality of life can be assessed using one of the following methods: telephone, self-administered, or replacement responders. Each strategy has its own set of advantages and disadvantages. Aside from the possibility of better responsiveness, specific measures have the advantage of being directly related to areas that clinicians usually investigate. For example, interviewer administered has a high response rate, few or no missing items, and few misinterpretation errors, but it involves a lot of resources, including interview training. It may also make people less reluctant to admit they have a problem. The telephone administration is similar to the interviewer-administered one, although it may limit the instrument combinations. However, when using a self-administered strategy, just a little amount of resources are used, which increases the chances of a poor response rate, missing items, and misunderstanding. In another strategy, termed replacement responders, stress for the target group is lessened but the perspective of the substitutes may be different from the target group [21].

4.3 Which HRQoL Instrument to use?

Certain factors are there to identify whether the instrument to measure HRQoL is good or bad. Some of them are listed as follows:

- **Time of measurement**: It should be clearly indicated whether one is measuring at a point in time or measuring a change over time? The goal of HRQoL measurement includes identifying between people who have better, moderate or worse HRQoL, *discriminative instrument,* and measuring to what extent the HRQoL of the people changed, *evaluative instrument*. In this regards, instrument and the characteristic features of the clients must be taken in to account before deciding which type of instrument measure the HRQoL.

- **The Validity of the instrument**: Validity refers to whether an instrument measures what it intends to measure. In this regard, the presence of the gold standard matters to use the given tool. To use validity when there is a gold standard instrument, one must determine using 'criterion validity'. If the results of an instrument fit the criterion standard, it is called genuine. When a shorter version of an instrument (the test) is used to predict the results of the full-length index, for example, criterion validity is applicable (the gold standard). Another example is predicting mortality using an HRQL instrument. Another example is predicting mortality using an HRQL instrument. In this case, the instrument will be valid to the extent that the questionnaire results explain variation in patient survival (the gold standard) (the test). Individual evaluations of physiological, physical, psychological, and social well-being are included in self-ratings of health, as are more extensive and longer assessments of general health views. Self-ratings of perceived health are a significant predictor of mortality [21, 22]. In the absence of a gold standard, HRQoL researchers adopt validation procedures from clinical and experimental psychologists who have struggled for years to determine whether questionnaires assessing intelligence, attitudes, and emotional function are measuring what they are supposed to measure. Content and construct validity are two types of validity that psychologists have introduced [21].

- **Interpretability:** The 'interpretability' of an HRQL metric is a final important feature. A discriminative tool may be used to determine if a given score indicates that a patient is functioning properly or has mild, moderate, or severe HRQL impairment. One can question whether a given change in score reflects a trivial, minor but significant, moderate, or major improvement or deterioration for an evaluative instrument [21].

5. The structure of health-related quality of life measures

Some HRQ0L measurements are as simple as asking the patient, "How is your quality of life?" [23]. This question can be asked in a straightforward or complex manner, with either option producing restricted results. HRQoL tools are often questionnaires with a number of elements or questions. Domains are made up of items (also sometimes called dimensions). The area of behavior or experience that is being measured is referred to as a domain or dimension. Mobility and self-care are two domains that can be combined to form physical function, sadness, anxiety, or well-being, which can then be combined to produce an emotional function domain. Because it comprises eight aspects rather than a single summative measure, the short form 36 (SF-36) is one of the finest ways for measuring HRQoL in chronic conditions. Physical functioning, Social functioning, Bodily pain, Role limitations caused by physical health problems (Role/physical), Role limitations caused by emotional problems (Role/emotional), Emotional well-being (Mental health), Energy/fatigue (Vitality), and General health perceptions are all evaluated by questions in the eight dimensions. These eight aspects can be summarized into two components: physical health component summary and mental health component summary. Physical functioning, role limitations due to physical health problems, bodily pain, and general health perception are included in the physical health component summary, whereas social functioning, role limitations due to mental health problems, and general health perception are included in the mental health component summary. Each of the eight dimensions expressly assesses the patients' quality of life, such as;

Physical Function (PF): The degree to which health restricts physical activities like walking, self-care, stair climbing, lifting, and workouts.

Role Physical (RF): The degree to which physical health interferes with work, such as completing fewer tasks and having difficulty executing activities.

Body Pain (BP): The severity of pain and how it affects one's ability to work.

Vitality (VT): is the difference between feeling energized and exhausted and worn out.

Social Functioning (SF): The degree to which physical or emotional difficulties obstruct social activity.

Emotional Role (RE): The degree to which emotional issues interfere with work, such as decreased time spent on activities and completing fewer tasks.

Mental Health (MH): General mental health, including depression, anxiety, behavioral-emotional control.

General Health (GH): The degree to which one can subjectively judge his or her health condition in comparison to that of a year ago, as well as the level of physical activity.

These eight components are added together to form overall HRQoL, allowing the level of HRQoL of patients/clients to be calculated. Each raw scale score was turned into a 0–100 scale after the score for each domain was obtained by adding each item under each domain. The overall HRQoL was then determined by multiplying each converted domain score by eight to get the overall HRQoL (number of domains). The higher the total score, the higher the quality of life; the lower the score, the poorer the quality of life. Scores of 45 poor/bad/low HRQoL, 46–65 moderate HRQoL, and > 65 relatively high HRQoL are used to interpret the final score for the total score [24, 25].

6. Predictors of health-related quality of life among patients with diabetes mellitus

From the study conducted among patients with diabetes mellitus on follow-up at one of the public specialized hospitals in Ethiopia, age, sex, marital status, educational status, smoking history, feeling of stigma, co-morbidity status, chronic complication and body mass index (BMI) were the potential predictors of HRQoL. The study indicated that, the overall HRQoL of patients with diabetes on follow-up at the study area was found to be moderate. General health, mental health, bodily pain and vitality were the most affected domains of HRQoL [24].

The study participants' overall HRQoL was found to have a transformed mean score of 50.318.1, with minimum and maximum scores of 16.4 and 79.1, respectively. The study participants had the highest (63.234.4) mean score in physical functioning and the lowest (30.222.9) mean score in the overall health domain among the eight domains of HRQoL. When the HRQoL was decomposed into domains, general health, mental health, bodily pain, and vitality all had a mean score below 50, indicating that they were the most affected (**Table 1**).

Principal component analysis (PCA) was also used to construct two-component HRQoL scores, with 66.77 percent of the total variance explained. The mental component score had a higher mean score (51.7716.72), with a maximum score of 80.75 (Appendices A-C).

According to this study, socio demographic status (age, sex, marital status, educational status), socio cultural status (feeling of stigmatized), behavioral factors (history of smoking) and clinical factors (co-morbidity status, chronic complication and body mass index are some of the predictors of health-related quality of life for patients living with diabetes mellitus [24]. Multiple linear regression was applied for the final model after controlling for the potential confounders and multicollinearity using variable inflation factor (VIF) (**Table 2**).

Domains of HRQoL, Overall HRQoL, PCS and MCS	Mean	SD	Minimum score (%)	Maximum score (%)
Physical Functioning (PF)	63.19	34.36	14.4	97.6
Social Functioning (SF)	56.04	30.13	12.9	98.6
Role limitation due to physical health (RP)	53.37	44.8	8.6	98.2
Role limitation due to emotional problem (RE)	52.71	45.82	6.97	98.6
Emotional wellbeing (MH)	49.84	8.02	20.0	72.0
Bodily Pain (BP)	48.60	11	12.5	80.0
Energy/Fatigue (VT)	48.47	7.78	20.0	75.0
General Health (GH)	30.21	22.95	7.3	95.0
Overall HRQoL	50.30	18.08	16.8	79.1
Physical Component Score (PCS)	48.84	21.87	10.0	87.5
Mental Component Score (MCS)	51.77	16.72	19.8	80.8

HRQoL: health-related quality of life; MCS: Mental Component Score; NSH: Nekemte Specialized Hospital; PCS: Physical Component Score.

Table 1.
The eight domains of HRQoL, the overall HRQoL and the two component scores of HRQoL with their mean score of diabetic patients at NSH, East Wollega, West Ethiopia, 15th April -5th June, 2019, (n = 215).

Residence, economic position, occupation, type of diabetes, drug regimen, and duration of diabetes mellitus were not statistically significant predictors of health-related quality of life, as shown in the table above.

Controlling for all other independent factors, the multiple linear regression model revealed that a unit increase in age would likely reduce health-related quality of life of diabetic patients by 0.25 (= − 0.25, 95% CI, −0.43.55, −0.07, p = 0.007). Other literatures also supported this finding [11, 26, 27]. This might be because of the physiological alteration of the patients as they got older. Older individuals are mostly limited in physical activities, coping with pain intensity and relief from pain [28]. However, findings from other parts of Ethiopia, South Africa and the Nordic countries were inconsistent with the current study result where age has no association with HRQoL [29–31].

Being male was positively associated with better HRQoL compared to their counter parts (β = 5.23, 95% CI, 1.10–9.36, p = 0.013). Literatures are inconsistently explaining in this regard [11, 12, 27, 32, 33]. This disagreement could be due to the gender impact as most of the time women are treated inferiorly. They are less autonomous in giving decision on behalf of their rights. Moreover, evidences showed that women were more likely affected by DM than males. Women also are more susceptible to the risk of central obesity when compared to men which in turn lead to the enhancement of the risk of complication of DM. This greatly reduces HRQoL of the clients [34]. As for marital status, being married was positively associated as it would likely increase the HRQoL by 5.30 units compared to those who were single controlling for all other independent variables (β = 5.30, 95% CI, 0.88–10.52. P = 0.046). The psychological stability and better social interaction when compared to those who are not in marriage would contribute for the association [29].

Regarding the educational level the respondents achieved, unable to read and write would likely decrease the HRQoL by 8.81 units (β = − 8.81, 95% CI,-14.88 to −2.82, P = 0.004) compared to those who achieved college and above after controlling for all other predictors.

The history of smoking was found to affect the HRQoL status of the patients with diabetes. Having smoking history would likely decrease the HRQoL by 9.03 units (β = − 9.03, 9 5% CI, −15.23- -4.69, P < 0.001) compared to their counter parts. Centers for Diseases Control and Prevention (CDC) and other study from USA indicated that Smokers are more likely to have central fat accumulation than non-smokers, and smoking is known to induce insulin resistance and compensatory insulin secretion responses, which could explain the increased risk of diabetes in those who smoke [35]. In the same way, feeling of stigmatized because of being patient with diabetes would likely decrease HRQoL by 5.25 units (β= − 5.25, 95% CI, −8.94 to −1.56, P = 0.005) compared to their counterparts controlling all other predictors. Multifaceted restrictions that the DM patients are facing, for example, the amount, type and timing of food consumed would attribute to the unsuitability of their social interaction. This in turn leads to the poorer HRQoL.

The absence of co morbid conditions and chronic complications related to diabetes mellitus increased HRQoL compared to their counter parts. In both cases, the absence of the condition would likely increase the HRQoL by about 6 units. As for BMI, the increase in one unit of BMI would likely decrease the HRQoL by 3.56 units (β= − 3.56, 95% CI,-6.94- -0.18, P = 0.009). This could be attributed that co morbid conditions are another challenge that could put the patients in disturbing conditions. Patients might seek healthcare for both or above diseases in which case they were emotionally diseased, the role due to emotional problem might be disputed. All the domains of HRQoL directly or indirectly would be affected. In another way,

Variables	Unstandardized coefficient		Standardized coefficient	95% CI		P-value
	B	SE	β	Lower	Upper	
(Constant)	69.41	10.31		49.16	89.74	0.000
Sex						
Female	1	1	1	1	1	1
Male	5.23	2.11	0.14	1.10	9.36	**0.013***
Age	-0.25	0.08	-0.20	-0.43	-0.07	**0.007***
Marital status						
Single	1	1	1	1	1	1
Married	5.30	2.69	0.11	0.88	10.52	**0.046***
Divorced	-4.60	5.26	-0.04	-14.98	5.78	0.38
Widowed	-4.07	3.42	-0.07	-10.81	2.67	0.24
Educational status						
Cannot read and write	-8.81	3.06	-0.19	-14.88	-2.82	**0.004***
Grade 1-8	-2.94	2.49	-0.07	-7.84	1.97	0.24
Grade 9-12	0.04	2.62	0.001	-5.13	5.22	0.98
College and above	1	1	1	1	1	1
Smoking history						
Yes	-9.03	2.66	-0.21	-15.23	-4.69	**0.000****
No	1	1	1	1	1	1
Feeling of stigmatized						
Yes	-5.25	1.89	-0.15	-8.94	-1.56	**0.005***
No	1	1	1	1	1	1
Co morbidity status						
Yes	1	1	1	1	1	1
No	6.05	2.18	0.16	1.78	10.33	**0.006***
Chronic complication status						
Yes	1	1	1	1	1	1
No	6.04	2.28	0.11	1.54	10.53	**0.009***
BMI	-3.56	1.71	-0.12	-6.94	-0.18	**0.040***
DM Duration	0.15	1.10	0.01	-2.02	2.33	0.89
Types of DM						
Type 1	1	1	1	1	1	1
Type 2	4.45	2.39	0.12	-0.24	9.17	0.064
Drug regimen						
Insulin only	1	1	1	1	1	1
OHA	-5.66	3.46	-0.16	-12.48	1.15	0.103
Both	-1.42	4.02	-0.02	-9.35	6.51	0.72

Dependent Variable: Overall health related quality of life, VIF: Variable Inflation Factor, VIF max = 4.16.
$^{*}P < 0.05$.
$^{**}P < 0.001$, Adjusted $R^2 = 0.536$, $F = 16.46$.

Table 2.
Multiple linear regression analysis of diabetic patients on follow up at NSH, East Wollega , West Ethiopia, 15th April -5th June, 2019, (n = 215).

those who developed chronic complications would also live under the double crisis. In one way, they felt unhappy about being patient with diabetes, and in another way, they would be under psychological, physical, emotional, social, and spiritual agony.

In conclusion, the present study identified that the HRQoL of patients with diabetes on follow-up at NSH was moderate. Domains of general health, mental health, bodily pain, and vitality were the most affected domains among the patients with diabetes. Sex, age, education status, marital status, history of smoking status, BMI, the feeling of stigma status, comorbidity status, and diabetic-related chronic complication status were predictors of HRQoL identified in this study.

It is recommended that health policy makers should give due attention for the overall HRQoL of the patients with diabetes on follow up at health institutions in addition to the existing treatment focused guidelines. Health care providers should also give emphasize to general health, mental health, bodily pain and vitality of the patients. Well scheduled, regular and continuous diabetic health education has to be provided as equally as important with the usual treatment and care for the patients. Respecting and understanding the patients' feeling has to be put first.

Moreover, health researchers should conduct further longitudinal studies with larger sample size in order to generalize the overall HRQoL of patients with diabetes at national level. Experimental and qualitative study design needs to be considered focusing the life style modification on patients with DM.

Annexes

A. Correlation matrix

Correlation Matrix									
	PF	**RP**	**VT**	**MH**	**BP**	**GH**	**RE**	**SF**	**Overall HRQoL**
PF	1.000								
RP	.631	1.000							
VT	.089	.127	1.000						
MH	.125	.208	.294	1.000					
BP	.043	.092	-.018	-.002	1.000				
GH	.455	.511	.133	.113	-.030	1.000			
RE	.380	.683	.071	.191	.034	.274	1.000		
SF	.590	.640	.166	.276	.042	.549	.327	1.000	
Overall HRQoL	.763	.916	.207	.301	.128	.637	.747	.765	1.000

B. Anti-image correlation (measures of sampling adequacy) of the fitted domains

	PF	**RP**	**VT**	**MH**	**GH**	**RE**	**SF**	**BP**	**Overall HRQoL**
PF	0.74								
RP		0.65							
VT			0.64						
MH				0.55					

	PF	RP	VT	MH	GH	RE	SF	BP	Overall HRQoL
GH					0.78				
RE						0.52			
SF							0.89		
BP								0.48	
Overall HRQoL									0.62

C. Table showing the rotated component matrix

Domains	Component 1	Component 2
Physical functioning	0.83	
Role physical	0.85	
Vitality		0.81
Metal Health		0.79
General health	0.75	
Social functioning		0.83
Role emotional		0.68
Bodily pain	0.48	

Author details

Bikila Regassa Feyisa
Wollega University, Nekemte, Ethiopia

*Address all correspondence to: bikregasa@gmail.com; bikilareg@wollegauniversity.edu.et

References

[1] American Diabetes Association. Standards of Medical Care for Patients. 2002;25(1):s33–49.

[2] Center for disease control and prevention. National Diabetes Fact Sheet , 2008.

[3] Trikkalinou A, Papazafiropoulou AK MA. World Journal of Diabetes. *Diabetol Metab Syndr.* 2017;8(4):120–71.

[4] Center for control and Prevention of diseases. Smoking and diabetes, 2014. Available from:https://www.cdc.gov/tobacco/data_statistics/sgr/50th-anniversary/pdfs/fs_smoking_diabetes_508.pdf.[cited 28Mar, 2019]

[5] Bommer C, Sagalova V, Heesemann E, Manne-goehler J, Atun R. Global Economic Burden of Diabetes in Adults : Projections From 2015 to 2030. 2020;41:963–70.

[6] International Diabetes Federation. IDF Diabetes Atlas : Global estimates of diabetes prevalence for 2017 and projections for 2045. *Diabetology & Metabolic Syndrome*. Elsevier B.V.; 2015. Available from: https://doi.org/10.1016/j.diabres.2018.02.023

[7] International Diabetes Federation. IDF DIABETES ATLAS. 2015.

[8] Al-shehri AH, Taha AZ, Bahnassy AA, Salah M. Health-related quality of life in type 2 diabetic patients. 2008;25(5):352–60.

[9] Kebede D, Alem A, Shibre T, Deyessa N. Health related quality of life (SF-36) survey in Butajira , rural Ethiopia : Normative data and evaluation of reliability and validity. 2004;289–97.

[10] Dinesh Khanna JT. Health-related Quality of Life- An Introduction. *Am J Manag Care*,. 2007;13(9):218–23.

[11] Goli M, Salarvand S, Dehvan F, Ghafouri H, Dalvand S. Health-Related Quality of Life in Iranian Patients with Thalassemia Major : A Systematic Review and Meta-Analysis. 2018;6(59): 8483–94.

[12] Sreedevi A, Cherkil S, Kuttikattu DS, Kamalamma L, Oldenburg B. Validation of WHOQOL-BREF in Malayalam and Determinants of Quality of Life Among People With Type 2 Diabetes in Kerala , India. 2016; 28(1s):62S–69S.

[13] Athanasia K. Papazafiropoulou, Florentia Bakomitrou, Aikaterini Trikallinou et al. Diabetes- dependent quality of life (ADDQOL) and affecting factors in patients with diabetes mellitus type 2 in Greece. *BioMed Central*; 2018;10(23):4–9.

[14] Hayek AA Al, Robert AA, Saeed A Al, Alzaid AA, Sabaan FS Al. Factors Associated with Health-Related Quality of Life among Saudi Patients with Type 2 Diabetes Mellitus : A Cross-Sectional Survey. 2014;38:220–9.

[15] Anderson BJ, Laffel LM, Domenger C, Danne T, Phillip M, Mazza C, et al. Factors Associated With Diabetes- Specific Health-Related Quality of Life in Youth With Type 1 Diabetes : *The Global TEENs Study*. 2017;40:1002–9.

[16] James P. Boyle, Amanda A. Honeycutt, K.M Venkat Narayan, Thomas J.Hoerger,Linda S.Geiss, Homg Chen, et al. Projection of Diabetes Burden Through 2050. *Diabetes Care* 2001;24(11):1936–40.

[17] Patrick D, Bergner M. Measurement of health status in the 1990s. *Annu Rev Public Health* 1990; 11:165-83.

[18] Patrick DL, Erickson P. Health Status and Health Policy: Quality of Life

in Health Care Evaluation and Resource Allocation. New York: Oxford University Press, 1993.

[19] Guyatt GH, Thompson PJ, Berman LC, et al. How should we measure function in patients with chronic heart and lung disease? *J Chron Dis* 1985; 38:517-24.

[20] Weinberg JE. Outcomes research, cost containment, and the fear of health care rationing. N *Engl J Med* 1990; 323: 1202-4.

[21] Gordon H Guyatt. Measuring health-related quality of life: General issues. *Can Respir J* Vol 4 No 3 May/ June 1997.

[22] Mossey J, Shapiro E. Self-rated health: a predictor of mortality among the elderly. *Am J Public Health* 1982; 72: 800-9.

[23] Torrance GW. Measurement of health state utilities for economic appraisal. *J Health Econ* 1986; 5:1-30.

[24] Feyisa BR, Yilma MT, Tolessa BE. Predictors of health-related quality of life among patients with diabetes on follow-up at Nekemte specialized Hospital, Western Ethiopia: a cross-sectional study. *BMJ Open,* 2020; 10: e036106. Doi: 10.1136/ bmjopen-2019-036106.

[25] W.Bani Issa. Evaluation of health related quality of life of Emirati people with diabetes: Integration of sociodemographic and disease related variables. *Eastern Mediterranian Health Journal*, 2011; 17(11):825-830.

[26] Kakhki AD, Abed Z. Health-related quality of life of diabetic patients Tehran. *Int J Endocrinol Metab* 2013;11: 1–6.

[27] Wegeberg A-ML, Meldgaard T, Hyldahl S, et al. Quantities of comorbidities affects physical, but not mental health related quality of life in type 1 diabetes with confirmed polyneuropathy. *World J Diabetes* 2019; 10:87–95.

[28] Daya R, Zbayat FJR. Effects of diabetes mellitus on health-related quality of life at a tertiary hospital in South Africa : A cross-sectional study. *Diabetol Metab Syndr* 2018;10:918–28.

[29] Wändell PE. Quality of life of patients with diabetes mellitus an overview of research in primary health care in the Nordic countries. *Diabetol Metab Syndr* 2018;10.

[30] Muze M, Hailu E, Woldemichael K, et al. Health related quality of life and its associated factors among diabetic patients attending diabetes clinic in Jimma university teaching hospital. *Diabetol Metab Syndr* 2018;10:7–11.

[31] Del Core MA, Ahn J, Wukich DK, et al. Gender differences on SF-36 patient-reported outcomes of diabetic foot disease. *Int J Low Extrem Wounds* 2018;17:1–7.

[32] Gillani SW, Ansari IA, Zaghloul HA, et al. Bridging glycated hemoglobin with quality of life and health state; a randomized case–control study among type 2 diabetes patients. *Diabetol Metab Syndr* 2018;10:1–10.

[33] Qin W, Blanchette JE, Murrock C. Exploring the relationship between lifestyle behaviors and health-related quality of life among older adults with diabetes. *Diabetes Educ* 2019;45:96–104.

[34] Tang TS, Brown MB, Funnell MM, et al. Social support, quality of life, and self-care behaviors among African Americans with type 2 diabetes. *Diabetes Educ* 2008;34:266–76.

[35] Ware JE, Sherbourne CD. The mos 36-item short-form health survey (SF-36). *Med Care* 1992;30:473–83.

Chapter 5

Quality of Life in Patients with Skin Disease and Their Cohabitants

Trinidad Montero-Vílchez, Manuel Sánchez-Díaz, Antonio Martínez-López and Salvador Arias-Santiago

Abstract

Health evaluation implies assess multidimensional aspects of a person's development, such as physical, social, psychological, and emotional features. It is important to consider all these factors to apply a needs-oriented each patient approach. Chronic skin diseases have a great impact on quality of life, even more than other chronic conditions. For example, hidradenitis suppurativa is estimated to impair quality of life more than cardiovascular disease, lung disease or endocrine diseases. Multiple tools have been developed to measure health-related quality of life in patient, being the Dermatology Life Quality Index (DLQI) the most used. Psoriasis, hidradenitis suppurativa, acne, atopic dermatitis and hair disorders are those with the greatest impact on patients' quality of life. Moreover, chronic skin conditions impair not only patients' quality of life, but also cohabitants. Nevertheless, there is scarce information regarding the impact on their cohabitants. So, the objective of this chapter is to review the literature to assess the psychological and social effects of dermatological conditions both on patients and cohabitants.

Keywords: Acne, Alopecia, Atopic Dermatitis, Cohabitants, Hidradenitis Suppurativa, Psoriasis, Quality of Life

1. Introduction

Health evaluation implies assess multidimensional facets of a person's development, such as physical, social, psychological and emotional aspects [1]. It is important to consider all these factors to apply a needs-oriented each patient approach. Chronic skin diseases have a great impact on quality of life, even more than other chronic conditions like asthma, epilepsy or diabetes [2]. Psoriasis, hidradenitis suppurativa, acne, atopic dermatitis and hair disorders are those with the greatest impact on patients' quality of life [2–4].

Multiple tools have been developed to measure health-related quality of life in patient, being the validated Dermatology Life Quality Index (DLQI) the most used. It evaluates the impact of skin symptoms of dermatological conditions and their treatment on patient's lives. The 10-item questionnaire covers the following aspects of patients' quality of life: symptoms and feelings, daily activities, leisure, work or school, personal relationships, and treatment. Each question is scored from 0 to 3 (not at all/not relevant (0), a little [1], a lot [2], and very much [3]) and

IntechOpen

reflects the extent to which the person's life quality is adversely affected by the skin condition. The total score ranges from 0 to 30, and higher score reflects a greater impairment in patients' life [5]. The DLQI punctuation is interpreted 0–1 = no effect at all; 2–5 = small effect; 6–10 = moderate effect; 11–20 = very large effect; 21–30 = extremely large effect [6]. There are also other scales to assess anxiety, depression or sexual dysfunction that are also uses to evaluate different aspects of patients' quality of life [6, 7]. The validated Hospital Anxiety and Depression Scale (HADS) is used to evaluate the prevalence of anxiety and depression. It is divided into two scales of seven items each. Scores equal or higher than 8 on the subscales are indicative of anxiety or depression [8]. The validated International Index of Erectile Function (IIEF-5) and the Female Sexual Function Index (FSFI-6) questionnaires are used to evaluate sexual dysfunction in men and women, respectively. Scores lower than 22 for IIEF-5 and lower than 20 are indicative of sexual dysfunction [9, 10]. Furthermore, to compare different diseases impact on quality of life or to compare several treatment improvements in patients' life, quality-adjusted life-year (QALYs) or global disability-adjusted life years (DALYs) are used [11, 12].

Chronic skin conditions impair not only patients' quality of life, but also cohabitants. In fact, it has been described caregiver burnout syndrome, expressing with stress, anxiety or depression what may impair people's life [13]. This means that the primary caregivers of a sick person are also affected by the disease. Although there is scarce information regarding the impact on cohabitants' quality of life, recently the Family Dermatology Life Quality Index (FDLQI) has been developed. It is a 10-item questionnaire that covers family member's perception of a certain specific impact on his/her quality of life over the last 1 month. Each item is scored on a four-point scale (0–3). The final scored is calculated by summing the scores of individual items and ranges from of 0 to 30. Higher total FDLQI scores indicate greater impairment of the family member's quality of life [14]. FDLQI could be interpreted similarly to DLQI: 0–1 = no effect at all; 2–5 = small effect; 6–10 = moderate effect; 11–20 = very large effect; 21–30 = extremely large effect.

The objective of this chapter is to review the literature to assess the psychological and social effects of dermatological conditions both on patients and cohabitants.

2. Material and methods

Search strategy. A literature search was performed using Medline, Scopus and Embase from conception to November 2020. The following search terms were used: ((Dermatology) OR (Skin diseases) OR (Alopecia) OR (Psoriasis) OR (Hidradenitis Suppurativa) OR (Acne) OR (Acne Inversa) OR (Atopic Dermatitis)) AND (Quality of Life).

Inclusion and exclusion criteria. The search was limited to: (i) human data, (ii) articles regarding impairment in quality of life in patients and cohabitants, (iii) articles written in English or Spanish. All types of epidemiological studies (clinical trials, cohort studies, case–control studies and cross-sectional studies) were included and analyzed. Reviews, guidelines, protocols, and conference abstracts were excluded. Skin conditions were selected regarding their high prevalence, their severity and their high impairment in quality of life. Psoriasis, hidradenitis suppurativa, atopic dermatitis, acne and alopecia were included. Only studies using validate scales to assess impairment in quality of life were included.

Study selection. Two researchers (TMV and MSD) independently reviewed the titles and abstracts of the articles obtained in the first search to assess relevant studies. The full texts of all articles meeting the inclusion criteria were reviewed, and their bibliographic references were checked for additional sources. The articles considered relevant by both researchers were included in the analysis. Disagreements about inclusion or exclusion of articles were subjected to discussion until a consensus was reached. If not reached, resolution was achieved by discussion with a third researcher (SAS).

Variables. The variables assessed were number of participants and cohabitants, assent tools used to evaluate quality of life, risk factors associated with impairment in cohabitants' quality of life, general impairment in patients' quality of life.

Target audience. Clinicians and research are the main audience of this review. Doctors should be aware to consider patients and cohabitant impairment in quality of life when making treatment decisions. Moreover, research should include validate measure of patients and cohabitants quality of life in their investigations.

2.1 Psoriasis

Psoriasis is a chronic, recurrent, multi-systemic inflammatory disease that mainly affects the skin and the joints [15]. It is a multifactorial disease caused by a combination of immunological imbalance, genetic associations and environmental factors [16]. Its prevalence around the word has been estimated from between 0.51% and 11.43% [17], being more frequent in countries more distant from the equator [18]. In Europe, psoriasis prevalence is about 1.3% [19]. Furthermore, its incidence is increasing over the years [19, 20]. It has a bimodal age of onset (16 to 22 and 57 to 60 years) [21] and it affects both sexes similarly [18].

Psoriasis is considered a major global health problem [22]. Although, the skin manifestations are commonly the only recognized symptoms of psoriasis [20], this disease is associated with multiple comorbidities such as arthritis, cardiovascular disease, metabolic syndrome, depression, anxiety or inflammatory bowel disease [23–26]. All of them contribute to increase the morbimortality in these patients. In fact, similar to many chronic inflammatory diseases, the risk of early mortality in patients with psoriasis is increased, especially due to cardiovascular events [27]. Likewise, the risk of mortality from cardiovascular disease is higher in patients with more severe psoriasis [28]. Patients with psoriasis are also at increased risk of mental problems. Rates of anxiety, depression and even suicide are increased in these patients [29]. Psoriasis can also influence the interpersonal and sexual health of people with psoriasis [30]. Psoriasis therefore impacts on physical, emotional, and social patient's life [20]. Moreover, the economic burden of psoriasis is high, as in Europe the annual total cost per patient is between 6,000-12,000€ [31].

Furthermore, psoriasis has a great impact on cohabitants' life [6, 7, 32]. The presence of psoriasis impaired the quality of life in almost 90% of the cohabitants. FDLQI scores of cohabitants are associated with the DLQI scores of the patients. Moreover, an increased body surface area affected, and the genital and scalp location were associated with a higher FDLQI score while FDLQI scores were lower for cohabitants with higher professional/university education [6]. Disease severity and duration impact negatively on cohabitants' quality of life, anxiety and depression [6, 32]. In addition, after getting psoriasis, a reduction in the frequency of sexual intercourse occurred in in more than 90% of the relationship and 40% of psoriasis partners suffer from sexual dysfunction [7, 32].

Multiple treatments are effective for treating psoriasis, including topical medications, phototherapy, oral systemic medications, and biologics [33]. Mild psoriasis can be treated with topical corticosteroids or corticosteroids plus vitamin D analogues. Moderate psoriasis needs to be treated with systemic treatments, such as methotrexate, acitretin or cyclosporine, or phototherapy. If psoriasis is severe or treatment-resistant, biologics are indicated. There is a wide range of biologics therapies for treating psoriasis: TNFα (etanercept, adalimumab, infliximab, certolizumab), IL12/23 inhibitors (ustekinumab), IL23 inhibitor (guselkumab, risankizumab, tildrakizumab), IL17 inhibitors (secukinumab, ixekizumab, brodalumab) [34]. The economic outcomes of these targeted treatments have been compared with non-targeted ones. The incremental benefits compared with no targeted treatment are, in descending order: ixekizumab 1.68 QALYs, brodalumab 1.64 QALYs, secukinumab 1.51 QALYs, ustekinumab 1.43 QALYs, infliximab 1.27 QALYs, adalimumab 1.15 QALYs, etanercept 0.97 QALYs, and apremilast 0.87 QALYs. Initial targeted treatment with IL-17 inhibitors seems to be the most effective treatment strategy for plaque psoriasis patients who have failed systemics [11].

2.2 Hidradenitis suppurativa

Hidradenitis suppurativa (HS) is a chronic, recurrent, debilitating inflammatory skin disease of the hair follicle that usually presents after puberty with painful, deep-seated inflamed lesions in the apocrine gland-bearing areas of the body, most commonly the axillae, inguinal and anogenital regions [35]. A prevalence rate of around 1% has been estimated [36], of 0.03–1% in Europe [37–39] and of 0.053% in the USA [40].

Its etiopathogenesis is still elusive and may be of pivotal importance in improving patients and relative's quality of life. Genetic susceptibility, smoking, obesity and hormonal disorders are major risk factors for the development of HS [41]. Moreover HS, has been associated with multiple physical comorbidities such as spondylarthritis, inflammatory bowel disease and increased cardiovascular risk [42, 43]. Moreover, HS impairs patients' mental health. It has been related to higher levels of depression, anxiety, worse quality of life, sexual dysfunction and a higher suicide risk [44–47]. HS also has consequences on social relationships and professional careers, as high rates of absenteeism and unemployment have been reported in HS patients [43]. For all these reasons, HS is a stigmatizing and disabling disease that greatly impairs physical, emotional, and social patient's life. Moreover, the economic burden of HS is high [48]. Direct medical costs due only to surgery are around £2,000 per patient per year in the UK [49]. Indirect costs, for expel associated with frequent and long-term absenteeism and disability, have also a great impact on the health system [50].

Moreover, HS has a great impact on cohabitants' life as they are involved in patients' caregiving [51–53]. A positive association between the Dermatology Life Quality Index (DLQI) and the Family Dermatology Life Quality Index (FDLQI) has been observed [52]. The most affected areas are emotional distress (depression, anxiety, embarrassment), social life and routine household expenditure [53]. In fact, patient's anxiety and depression and higher score for negative affectivity are associated with a lower quality of life in their cohabitants [52]. Disease severity also impairs both patients and cohabitants life due to skin symptoms (disease duration, pain, more involved locations), the need of continuous care and more unpleasant treatments and a higher economic expenditure [51]. In addition, a great impact is found in partners or husband/wife compared with parents, leading to a potential effect on the couple relationships [51]. In fact, patient sexual dysfunction greatly impairs cohabitant's quality of life [52]. On the other hand, higher educational level and an early diagnosis and treatment have a positive impact on patients and their partners' life [51–53].

HS therapy is often challenging and requires the combination of medical and surgical treatments [54, 55]. Medical treatment of mild disease consists in topical clindamycin 1% solution/gel twice a day for 12 weeks or, for a more widespread disease, tetracycline 500 mg daily for 4 months. If patient do not respond or for moderate-to-severe disease, clindamycin 300 mg with rifampicin 600 mg daily for

10 weeks would be considered [56]. Adalimumab, a monoclonal antibody against tumor necrosis factor-α, is the only biologic agent currently available for treating moderate to severe HS, but a primary or secondary lack of response has been observed in some patients [57]. New insights into the pathogenesis of HS reveal an inflammatory cytokine profile including elevated levels of (TNF)-α, interleukin (IL)-1ß, IL-17 or interferon (IFN)-γ and other biologic treatments such as bermekimab, bimekizumab, brodalumab, guselkumab, risankizumab or secukinumab are being tested in clinical trials [58]. There is scarce evidence regarding cost-effectiveness therapies in HS. It has been estimated that the incremental cost-effectiveness ratio for adalimumab versus standard care was around £30,000 per QALY gained [59]. Nevertheless, it cost-effectiveness was highly susceptible to the health states' utility values, the treatment discontinuation and the resource utilization [60].

2.3 Acne

Acne vulgaris is a chronic inflammatory disease of the pilosebaceous unit that usually presents at adolescence with comedones (blackheads and whiteheads), papules, pustules, nodules, cysts and scars. The most affected areas corresponds to the highest density of pilosebaceous units (face, neck, upper chest, shoulders, and back) [61]. It is a prevalent condition that involves 85% of adolescents and 6–10% of the general population [62].

Acne is a multifactorial disease resulting from androgen-induced disturbed sebaceous gland activity associated with increased sebum production and alterations in sebum fatty acid composition, altered keratinisation, inflammation, *Propionibacterium acnes* colonization of hair follicles and dysfunction of the innate and adaptive immunity [63]. Genetic susceptibility, air pollution, aggressive skincare products, corticosteroids and hormonal products are risk factors to develop acne. The role of nutrition in acne pathogenesis is still controversial [64]. Acne is associated with physical disability due to painful skin lesions. Moreover, it usually affects visible areas, with risk of permanent scarring and aesthetic consequences. In fact, acne is associated with high rates of anxiety, depression and even suicide [65, 66]. People with acne are also more prone to have social phobia [67].

Acne not only impairs patients' life but also their cohabitants. More than 90% of people leaving with acne patients have impaired their quality of life. A positive correlation between FDLQI in cohabitants and DLQI in patients is observed. Furthermore, patients' level of depression and anxiety are also associated with their cohabitants' [68].

Acne treatment is based on disease severity, patient preference, site of involvement, age of the patient and tolerability. Topical therapies may be used as monotherapy, in combination with other topical agents or in combination with oral agents in both initial control and maintenance. The most employed topical products are benzoyl peroxide, salicylic acid, antibiotics, combination antibiotics with benzoyl peroxide, retinoids, retinoid with benzoyl peroxide, retinoid with antibiotic, azelaic acid, and sulfone agents. Systemic antibiotics are used in moderate to severe inflammatory acne and should be used in combination with a topical retinoid and benzoyl peroxide. Tetracycline, mainly doxycycline and minocycline, are the most effective antibiotics. Oral contraceptives can improve acne for many women, mainly in those with clinical or laboratory signs of hyperandrogenism. Oral isotretinoin is indicated for severe acne or moderate treatment-resistant acne [69]. The effectiveness and cost effectiveness of isotretinoin are well proven as its cost per QALY of £898 ($US 13 74) is affordable [70]. Dermatologist treatment appears cost-effective related to producing additional QALYs at a cost of $40,000 per QALY gained [71].

2.4 Atopic dermatitis

Atopic dermatitis (AD) is a common and chronic inflammatory skin disease. It is characterized by recurrent eczematous lesions and intense itch which develop in people of all ages and ethnicities. The prevalence of AD has been estimated around 12% in children and 7% in adults in United States [72]. It is considered the leading non-fatal health burden attributable to skin diseases [73]. The etiopathogenesis of AD is not completely understood. However, most studies agree that skin barrier dysfunction and immune dysregulation play a key role in the development of AD [74, 75]. Genetic polymorphisms in the filaggrin gene, which encode a major structural protein in the stratum corneum, upregulation of Th2 cytokines, such as IL-4 and IL-13, changes in the skin microbiome and altered lipid composition are thought to be responsible for the appearance of pruritus and skin lesions in patients suffering from AD [75–78].

AD is frequently associated with food allergy, asthma and rhinitis, which is also known as the "atopic march". This concept refers to the propensity for AD to begin early in life and be followed by the serial incidence of food allergy, asthma, and hay fever [79]. Other associated conditions include eosinophilic esophagitis [80], allergic contact dermatitis [81], cardiovascular disease [82] and infections [83, 84].

Skin lesions and severe symptomatology, including severe itch and skin pain, contribute to an impaired quality of life in patients suffering from AD. Psychosocial distress, stigma, sleep disturbance avoidance of social interaction are consequences of AD [85]. Significantly poorer dermatology-related quality of life scores have been found in patients with AD: higher DLQI [86] and Children's DLQI [87], greater Skindex affectation [88] and itch-related quality of life [89]. Different general quality of life scores are also affected in patients with AD [86, 87, 89]. Furthermore, the impact on quality of life is not restricted to the patient itself, but also affects to their cohabitants. It has been shown that parents of children with AD have lower quality-of-life scores [90–92] and that AD influences marital conflicts [93]. Regarding the sexual health, there is evidence that AD have a strong impact in sexual behavior. The involvement of visible areas and sensual areas leads to lower quality of life indexes and higher burden scores in patients with AD [94]. Moreover, people with more severe AD have a greater impact on sexuality [94, 95].

Given its high burden, AD have been associated with high QALY loss, even higher than autoimmune disorders, diabetes, food allergy and heart disease in both males and female [96]. Moreover, six-dimensional health state short form (SF-6D) score, an utility score which ranges from 0 (worst health) to 1 (best health) was estimated to 0.63 in severe AD. This was lower than SF-6D in high blood pressure (0.63), diabetes (0.65) and similar to anxiety, depression and heart disease (0.63) [96].

The treatment of AD follows a stepwise approach that is tailored according to disease severity and extension [85, 97]. Patient's education and basic skin care must be carried out in all patients, including those without active skin lesions. It consists of the frequent application of skin moisturizers, warm baths or showers using non-soap cleansers and avoidance of skin irritants. For mild and localized disease, treatment involves the use of topical corticosteroids (TCS) and topical calcineurin inhibitors (TCI). For moderate-to-severe and extensive disease, phototherapy or systemic drugs are indicated. Systemic immunosuppressants, such as cyclosporine, methotrexate, azathioprine and mycophenolate mofetil can be used [75, 85]. Dupilumab, a monoclonal antibody which acts as a targeted therapy for AD, is currently the most effective therapy por severe AD. It acts through the blockage of the IL-4 receptor alpha-chain [85, 98]. Emerging therapies include anti IL-13 and anti IL-31 antibodies, JAK inhibitors, and inhibitors of PDE-4 [85, 98].

Finally, AD places a high financial burden on patients, families and society through direct medical costs and decreased productivity. Taking this into account, a conservative estimate of the annual costs of atopic dermatitis in the United States (2015) is $5.297 billion [99]. Regarding the current development of novel treatments, which involve higher costs [100], these costs is likely to increase over the time.

2.5 Alopecia

Alopecia is a heterogeneous group of common skin disorders. This group can be divided into two minor groups: a) Non-cicatricial alopecia: Follicular epithelium is not replaced by connective tissue, so it is potentially reversible; b) Cicatricial alopecia: Follicular epithelium is replaced by connective tissue, so it is assumed that permanent injury of the follicular stem cell region has occurred.

2.5.1 Non-cicatricial alopecia

Many different skin conditions can be classified into this category. Most common and most representative non-cicatricial alopecia will be reviewed below.

2.5.1.1 Androgenetic Alopecia (AGA)

AGA is an androgen-dependent hereditary disorder resulting from the conversion of scalp terminal hairs into miniaturized vellus hairs in a characteristic pattern. Androgens act on the epithelial cells of genetically susceptible hair follicles in androgen-dependent areas, leading to follicular miniaturization [101]. Its frequency and severity increase with age, with at least 80% of Caucasian men and 50% of women showing signs of AGA by age 70 years [102, 103]. In male pattern hair loss, there is a progressive loss of hair in the frontal and bitemporal line, and also in the vertex. In the female pattern hair loss, the frontal hairline is spared with a diffuse central thinning of the crown.

In some studies, AGA has associated to age and family history of AGA. Moreover, some factors related to metabolic syndrome have also been related to AGA in both genders: Hypertension, diabetes mellitus and waist circumference [104].

As AGA is frequent and affects a visible area such as the scalp, it can lead to a significant impairment in the quality of life and social inhibition in patients. There is evidence of the impairment in quality-of-life scores in both males and female suffering from AGA: DLQI [105–107], Hairdex scale [105] and Skindex-29 scale [106]. Moreover, AGA has a negative impact on sexual function in premenopausal women, reflected in a decreased FSFI compared to healthy females [108].

Only two therapeutic agents have been approved by the Food and Drug Administration and European Medicines Agency for the treatment of AGA: Topical minoxidil (in both males and females), and oral finasteride (in males) [109]. Minoxidil was first introduced as an oral treatment for severe hypertension in the 1970s [110]. When hypertrichosis was observed as a side effect of this medication, both topical and oral formulations of minoxidil were developed to treat alopecia. Minoxidil changes the micro-environment of the hair follicle, inducing a prolonged anagen phase and increased hair growth. Most common presentations of topical minoxidil include 2% and 5% lotions which are applied 1 ml/12 hours. Although oral minoxidil seems to be effective to treat AGA, it is not yet approved [111]. Oral finasteride is approved for AGA in men with a dosage of 1 mg/24 hours. It acts through the inhibition of 5-alpha reductase and is effective and safe [109] in the treatment of AGA.

2.5.1.2 Alopecia Areata (AA)

AA is a common inflammatory hair loss, characterized by an autoimmune-mediated hair follicle destruction, due to the upregulation of inflammatory pathways. The lifetime incidence of AA is approximately 2% worldwide [112]. The etiology is still not fully understood, but the loss of immune privilege in the hair follicle seems to play a crucial role in the development of AA [113]. Clinical features of AA vary from the appearance of small, well-circumscribed patches of hair loss to a complete absence of body and scalp hair.

As AA is an autoimmune disorder, patients suffering from AA have a higher risk of developing autoimmune diseases: thyroid disorders [112, 114], with an incidence in AA between 2,3-14,6%; diabetes mellitus, with an incidence in AA between 0,4-11,1% [115]; and vitiligo, with an incidence in AA between 1,8-7,0% [115] are some of the most common. AA have also been associated with atopic diseases, metabolic syndrome, Helicobacter Pylori infection, and vitamin D deficiency [116]. Moreover, a 66–74% of lifetime prevalence of psychiatric disorders have been reported in AA patients, with a 38–39% lifetime prevalence of depression and a 39–62% prevalence of generalized anxiety disorder [117–120].

Regarding the quality of life in people suffering from AA, there is increasing evidence of the strong impact of AA in quality-of-life scores, which affects up to 76.7% of children and 77.6% of adults [121]. Impairments in DLQI as well as in alopecia specific scores have been reported [115, 121, 122]. Role-emotional, mental health and vitality domains seem to be the most affected [121]. Moreover, scalp involvement, anxiety and depression have a negative impact on the quality of life of patients with AA [121]. AA also impacts on sexual quality of life [123]. One study showed that both males and females suffering from AA had decreased sexual quality of life with low Sexual Quality of Life for Females (SQOL-F) and Sexual Quality of Life for Males (SQOL-M) scores. In this study, men strongly identified with the statement "I fell anxious" and women with the statement "I feel embarrassed".

Preliminary outcomes of a research conducted in the Hospital Virgen de las Nieves (Granada, Spain), which were presented at the national congress of the Spanish Dermatology Academy showed also a significant burden in cohabitants of patients with AA. Cohabitants of patients with AA had high FDLQI scores, which correlated to DLQI from patients. Anxiety in cohabitants also showed correlation with the time of evolution of the disease [124].

There are different therapeutic options for AA, depending on the age of the patient and the extension of the disease. Briefly, in adult patients suffering from isolated patches of hair loss or less than 25% of scalp hair loss are the best candidates to therapy with intralesional injections of potent corticosteroids (such as triamcinolone). In the case of adult patients who refuse the injections and children, potent topical corticosteroids (betamethasone, clobetasol) are considered the first-line therapy. An alternative for mild cases is the use of topical anthralin. When AA is extensive, systemic drugs are recommended. Systemic corticosteroids taken in low doses can be effective but involve serious long-term adverse events. Other systemic immunosuppressive agents can be useful in AA: methotrexate or azathioprine. JAK inhibitors (tofacitinib, baricitinib) are novel promising therapies for severe cases of AA [125, 126].

2.5.2 Cicatricial alopecia

A wide variety of diseases can be classified into this group, both primary skin diseases and secondary cicatricial alopecia. Given that most of cicatricial alopecia are relatively uncommon, there is scarce evidence regarding their comorbidities and their treatment. Moreover, almost any studies report data about the impairment in quality of life associated with these skin disorders.

Few studies address the issue of quality of life in patients with Frontal Fibrosing Alopecia (FFA) [127]. FFA is a cicatricial alopecia, typically appearing in post-menopausal woman, characterized by slowly progression of hair loss in the frontal, temporal or frontotemporal scalp and eyebrows. Hair follicles show perifollicular erythema and scale. Patients with FFA have been found to show impairments in DLQI, and anxiety and depression scores [127].

Preliminary outcomes of a research conducted in the Hospital Virgen de las Nieves (Granada, Spain), which were presented at the national congress of the Spanish Dermatology Academy showed a significant burden in cohabitants of patients with FFA. Cohabitants of patients with FFA had high FDLQ) scores, which correlated to DLQI from patients. Anxiety in cohabitants also showed correlation with the time of evolution of the disease. However, the impact on the quality of life in cohabitants of patients with FFA was lower than the impact on the cohabitants of patients with AA [124].

3. Discussion

Skin diseases have a great impact on patients and cohabitants quality of life. Clinicians should be aware of this issue so they can provide an individualized medicine, targeting not only the visible symptoms of the disease but also the impact on quality of life. Researchers should also include quality of life impairment scales for patients and cohabitants to measure the effectiveness of treatments. Universal scales are needed to homogenize results. Further research regarding skin conditions should include the impact of both patients and cohabitants' quality of life assessed by validate scales. Moreover, healthcare policy should also consider not also patients' needs but also cohabitants'.

The most common tools to assess impairment in quality of life were the DLQI (for patients) and the FDLQI (for cohabitants), **Table 1**. HS and psoriasis are the diseases that have a greater impact on patients and cohabitant quality of life. The media DLQI scores for HS was 13.34 points and the media FDLQI was 9.76 points [51–53]. Psoriatic patients reported a media of 10.79 points in the DLQI and their cohabitants reported a media of 12.8 points in the FDLQI [6, 7, 32]. The greater impairment of this disease could be explained because of the symptoms, chronicity and comorbidities associated. The clinical manifestations of HS cause pain, itching, malodor and suppuration, among other symptoms, which make life difficult for patients [35]. Pain is one of the most important problems in patients with HS, usually related to the inflammation of the nodules. Psoriatic plaques are also associated with itching and pain what cause an important physical burden in patients [15]. The lesions of these disease frequently appear on the genital area, having an impact on sexual life [15, 35]. The sexual impairment could also explain the great cohabitants impairment of quality of life [6, 52], apart from the chronicity of this disease and the caregiver burnout syndrome. The following disease with higher points in the DLQI was AD (media of 10.78) [86, 87, 89]. This could also be explained because of the itching and the sleep disorder associated with this disease [79]. Acne and alopecia were scored with the lowest rate quality of life impairment. Acne patients scored a media of 7.56 points in the DLQI and their cohabitants a media of 6.46 in the FDLQI [68]. This could be explained because it is a disease that usually happens in adolescent and it is temporary [65]. Alopecia patients recorded a media of 6.1 points in the DLQI and their cohabitants a media of 6.13 points [124]. This might be explained because they are not usually associated with other symptoms and

Disease	Article	Number of patients/ cohabitants included	Assessment tools used to evaluate quality of life	Patients	Cohabitant	Risk factor associated with impairment in cohabitants' quality of life	General impairment in patients' quality of life
Psoriasis	Martinez-Garcia E et al. 2014	34/49	DLQI	12 (range 1–28)	—	Negative factors: DLQI, marital status, cohabitants' anxiety, severe psoriasis, a long disease duration, genital and scalp location. Protective factors: Higher professional/university education	Increased risk of other diseases: arthritis, cardiovascular disease, metabolic syndrome, inflammatory bowel disease. Increased risk of mental problems: anxiety, depression, suicide. Impaired social life: interpersonal and sexual health., economic burden.
			FDLQI	—	8.82 (range 0–30)		
			IIEF-5/ FSFI-6 (sexual dysfunction, %)	79.1% females, 19.1% males	54.5% females, 59.2% males		
	Halioua, B et al. 2020	184/184	DLQI	9.57 (6.35 SD)	—	Negative factors: patients' quality of life, cohabitants' mental health, patient disease severity	
			FDLQI	—	16.78 (9.96 SD)		
Hidradenitis suppurativa	Ramos-Alejos-Pita C et al. 2020	27/27	DLQI	13.88 (SD 9.53)	—	Negative factors: patients' BMI, IHS4, impairment in patients' quality of life, patients' negative affectivity, patients' depression, sexual dysfunction, partners' sexual dysfunction	Physical comorbidities: spondylarthritis, inflammatory bowel disease and increased cardiovascular risk. Mental health: depression, anxiety, suicide. Impaired social life: sexual dysfunction, high rates of absenteeism and unemployment, economic burden
			FDLQI	—	10.48 (SD 7.76)		
			IIEF-5/ FSFI-6 (sexual dysfunction)	18.26 (SD 6.28)	20.82 (SD 6.51)		
	Wlodarek K et al. 2020	50/50	FDLQI	—	8.7 (SD 6.8)	Negative factors: patient's and partner's age, Hurley stage, HSSI	
	Marasca C et al. 2020	35/70	DLQI	12.8 (SD 4.48)	—	Negative factors: DLQI, Hurley stage, partner relationship Protective factors: Higher professional/university education	
			FDLQI	—	10.11 (range 0–19)		

Disease	Article	Number of patients/ cohabitants included	Assessment tools used to evaluate quality of life	Patients	Cohabitant	Risk factor associated with impairment in cohabitants' quality of life	General impairment in patients' quality of life
Acne	Martinez-Garcia E et al. 2014	62/66	DLQI	7.56 (range 0–29)	—	Negative factors: impairment in patients' quality of life, acne duration, cohabitant's anxiety level.	Physical disability: painful lesions. Mental health: high rates of anxiety, depression and suicide. Impaired social life: aesthetic consequences, social phobia.
			FDLQI	—	6.46 (range 0–26		
Atopic dermatitis	Xu X et al. 2019	559 / 559	IDQOL	8.76 (SD 2.6)	—	Negative factors: Higher CDLQI and IDQOL, severity of the disease, and children's age.	Age and severity of the disease was related to lower quality of life in children. Patients have an increased risk of food allergies, asthma, hay fever, eosinophilic esophagitis, allergic contact dermatitis, cardiovascular disease and infections.
			CDLQI	8.76 (SD 2.2)	—		
			RAND-36	—	38.52 (SD 7.16)		
	Ezzedine K et al. 2020	399 / 399	CDLQI	8.7 (SD 7.1)	—	Negative factors: Children's age, higher CDLQI and DLQI, shorter disease duration, younber parents.	
			DLQI	12.8 (SD 11.1)	—		
			ABS-F	—	10.0 (SD 8.0)		
	Gieler U et al. 2017	64 / 64	GDS, QPCAE.	—	.	Negative factor: Being a single mother of a child with atopic dermatitis led to higher perceived stress in the family and less life-satisfaction when compared to mothers with partners.	
	Jang HJ et al. 2016	78 / 78	DFI	—	—	Negative factors: Severity of the disease, children's female gender, parent's stress and negative affect led to lower family quality of life.	

Disease	Article	Number of patients/ cohabitants included	Assessment tools used to evaluate quality of life	Patients	Cohabitant	Risk factor associated with impairment in cohabitants' quality of life	General impairment in patients' quality of life
Alopecia Areata	Arias-Santiago S et al. 2020 (preliminary outcomes)	16 / 16	DLQI	6.5	—	Negative factors: The evolution time of the diseases led to higher anxiety and depression scores in cohabitants. Higher FDLQI correlates to higher anxiety and depression scores	Patients with AA have higher risk of thyroid disorders, diabetes mellitus, vitiligo, atopic diseases, metabolic syndrome, Helicobacter Pylori infection, and vitamin D deficiency. There is a 66–74% of lifetime prevalence of psychiatric disorders (depression and prevalence of generalized anxiety disorder).
			FDLQI	—	7.25 (SD 4.89)		
Frontal Fibrosing Alopecia	Arias-Santiago S et al. 2020 (preliminary outcomes)	15 / 15	DLQI	5,7	—	Negative factors: The evolution time of the diseases led to higher anxiety and depression scores in cohabitants. Higher FDLQI correlates to higher anxiety and depression scores	There is scarce evidence regarding the comorbidities of FFA. Patients with FFA have been found to show impairments in DLQI, and anxiety and depression scores.
			FDLQI	—	5		

ABS-F: Atopic dermatitis Burden Scale-Family; CDLQI: Children's Dermatology Quality of Life Index; DFI: Dermatitis Family Impact questionnaire; DLQI, Dermatology Life Quality Index; FDLQI, Family Dermatology Life Quality Index; GDS: General Depression Scale; HSSI, Hidradenitis Suppurativa Severity Index; IDQOL: Infant's dermatitis quality of life; IIEF-5, International Index of Erectile Function; QPCAE: Questionnaire for Parent so Children with Atopic Eczema; SFI-6, Female Sexual Function Index;.

Table 1.
Articles regarding quality-of-life impairment in patients with skin diseases and cohabitants.

some types of alopecia, such as alopecia areata, are not chronic and patients can be completely recovered from its disease [125].

Regarding psychological impact of patients and cohabitants, HADS-A and HADS-D are the most frequent scales used, **Table 2**. The highest rates of patient's anxiety are reported for HS (9.51) and psoriasis (8.82), followed by frontal fibrosing alopecia (7.5), acne (6.9) and alopecia areata (6.6). The highest rates of cohabitants

Disease	Article	Number of patients/ cohabitants included	Assessment tools used to evaluate quality of life	Patients	Cohabitant
Psoriasis	Martinez-Garcia E et al. 2014	34/49	HADS-Anxiety	8.82 (range 1–18)	8.06 (range 0–16)
			HADS-Depression	6.15 (range 0–19)	4.73 (range 0–14)
			Rosenberg's Self-Esteem Questionnaire (<15, %)	78.2% females, 31.8% males	56.6% females, 40.8% males
	Halioua, B et al. 2020	184/184	MCS-12	41.94 (SD 10.35)	45.50 (SD 11.00)
			PSC-12	45.57 (SD 5.63)	44.92 (SD 5.75)
	Alariny AF et al. 2019	120/120	HADS-A (> 7, %)	69.1% females, 39.1% males	63.6% females, 51% males
			HADS-D (> 7, %)	39.1% females, 21.8% males	45.5% females, 34.7% males
Hidradenitis suppurativa	Ramos-Alejos-Pita C et al. 2020	27/27	HADS-Anxiety	9.51 (SD 4.89)	7.22 (SD 4.20)
			HADS-Depression	7.70 (SD 5.11)	5.14 (SD 4.52)
Atopic Dermatitis	Gieler U et al. 2017	64 / 64	SSQ, SWLS.	—	—
	Jang HJ et al. 2016	78 / 78	SWLS, PANAS	—	—
Acne	Martinez-Garcia E et al. 2014	62/66	HADS-A	6.29 (range 0–15)	6.91 (range 1–19)
			HADS-D	2.47 (range 0–11)	4.23 (range 0–16)
Alopecia Areata	Arias-Santiago S et al. 2020 (preliminary outcomes)	16 16	HADS - Anxiety	6.6	6.5
			HADS - Depression	4.9	6
Frontal Fibrosing Alopecia	Arias-Santiago S et al. 2020 (preliminary outcomes)	15 / 15	HADS - Anxiety	7.5	4.5
			HADS - Depression	4.1	3

HADS, Hospital Anxiety and Depression Scale; MCS-12, Mental Health Subscale; PANAS: Positive Affect and Negative Affect Schedule; PCS-12, Physical Health Subscale; SWLS: Satisfaction With Life Score; SSC: Short Stress Questionnaire.

Table 2.
Articles regarding psychological impairment in patients with skin diseases and cohabitants.

anxiety are reported for psoriasis (8.06), followed by HS (7.22), acne (6.91), alopecia areata (6.5) and frontal fibrosing alopecia (4.5). Depression was rated lower than anxiety in all diseases. Patients reported the highest rates for HADS-Depression in HS (7.7) and psoriasis (6.15), followed by alopecia areata (4.9), frontal fibrosing alopecia (4.1) and acne (2.47). Cohabitants reported the highest rates for HADS-Depression in alopecia areata [6], HS (5.14), psoriasis (4.73), acne (4.23) and frontal fibrosing alopecia. Up to our knowledge, there are no reports regarding the impact of AD in cohabitants anxiety and depression. In agreement with DLQI and FDLQI scores, psoriasis and HS are the diseases that have the greatest impact on patients and cohabitants anxiety [6, 7, 32, 51–53]. Regarding depression, patients' reports are in agreement with anxiety and DLQI scores. Nevertheless, cohabitants reported the highest scores for anxiety in alopecia areata [124]. This might be due because most alopecia areata patients are children and their hair loss negatively affect their parent's psycho [112].

4. Conclusion

Since skin lesions are visible and can generate unpleasant sensations, such as itching or pain, skin diseases are a major cause of decreased quality of life. In addition, the involvement of areas with a high emotional burden, such as the genital area, scalp o facial area can lead to social inhibition, anxiety and depression. Studies focused on the evaluation of the quality of life of patients and cohabitants with skin diseases and their co-habitants are necessary to objectify the great burden they bear. Therefore, it seems necessary to make a comprehensive approach to skin diseases, taking into account not only the medical aspect, but also the emotional and the quality of life of both patients and cohabitants.

The holistic approach of the skin disease requires the complete evaluation of patients and cohabitants, from the biological, psychological and social point of view. This approach should include specific evaluations of quality of life and related disorders in all patients and cohabitants, which will lead to a better quality of the health of the populations. Moreover, therapeutic methods aimed at improving the quality of life such as patient schools, cognitive-behavioral strategies or mindfulness should be implemented in the daily clinical practice to treat not only the biologic, but also the social and psychologic manifestations of skin diseases.

Conflict of interest

The authors have no conflict of interest to declare.

Funding

None.

Author details

Trinidad Montero-Vílchez[1,2], Manuel Sánchez-Díaz[1,2], Antonio Martínez-López[1,2] and Salvador Arias-Santiago[1,2,3]*

1 Dermatology Department, Hospital Universitario Virgen de las Nieves, Granada, Spain

2 Instituto de Investigación Biosanitaria IBS, Granada, Spain

3 Dermatology Department, Faculty of Medicine, University of Granada, Granada, Spain

*Address all correspondence to: salvadorarias@ugr.es; salvadorarias@hotmail.es

References

[1] Buendia-Eisman A, Arias-Santiago S. Quality of life and questionnaires in dermatology. *Actas Dermosifiliogr*. 2016;**107**:449-50.

[2] Mallon E, Newton JN, Klassen A, Stewart-Brown SL, Ryan TJ, Finlay AY. The quality of life in acne: a comparison with general medical conditions using generic questionnaires. *Br J Dermatol*. 1999;**140**:672-6.

[3] Matusiak L. Profound consequences of hidradenitis suppurativa: a review. *Br J Dermatol*. 2020;**183**:e171-e7.

[4] Sanclemente G, Burgos C, Nova J, Hernandez F, Gonzalez C, Reyes MI, et al. The impact of skin diseases on quality of life: A multicenter study. *Actas Dermosifiliogr*. 2017;**108**:244-52.

[5] Finlay AY, Khan GK. Dermatology Life Quality Index (DLQI)--a simple practical measure for routine clinical use. *Clin Exp Dermatol*. 1994;**19**:210-6.

[6] Martinez-Garcia E, Arias-Santiago S, Valenzuela-Salas I, Garrido-Colmenero C, Garcia-Mellado V, Buendia-Eisman A. Quality of life in persons living with psoriasis patients. *J Am Acad Dermatol*. 2014;**71**:302-7.

[7] Alariny AF, Farid CI, Elweshahi HM, Abbood SS. Psychological and Sexual Consequences of Psoriasis Vulgaris on Patients and Their Partners. *J Sex Med*. 2019;**16**:1900-11.

[8] Zigmond AS, Snaith RP. The hospital anxiety and depression scale. *Acta Psychiatr Scand*. 1983;**67**:361-70.

[9] Rosen RC, Cappelleri JC, Smith MD, Lipsky J, Pena BM. Development and evaluation of an abridged, 5-item version of the International Index of Erectile Function (IIEF-5) as a diagnostic tool for erectile dysfunction. *Int J Impot Res*. 1999;**11**:319-26.

[10] Isidori AM, Pozza C, Esposito K, Giugliano D, Morano S, Vignozzi L, et al. Development and validation of a 6-item version of the female sexual function index (FSFI) as a diagnostic tool for female sexual dysfunction. *J Sex Med*. 2010;**7**:1139-46.

[11] Hendrix N, Ollendorf DA, Chapman RH, Loos A, Liu S, Kumar V, et al. Cost-Effectiveness of Targeted Pharmacotherapy for Moderate to Severe Plaque Psoriasis. *J Manag Care Spec Pharm*. 2018;**24**:1210-7.

[12] Villasante Fricke AC, Miteva M. Epidemiology and burden of alopecia areata: a systematic review. *Clin Cosmet Investig Dermatol*. 2015;**8**:397-403.

[13] Alves LCS, Monteiro DQ, Bento SR, Hayashi VD, Pelegrini LNC, Vale FAC. Burnout syndrome in informal caregivers of older adults with dementia: A systematic review. *Dement Neuropsychol*. 2019;**13**:415-21.

[14] Basra MK, Sue-Ho R, Finlay AY. The Family Dermatology Life Quality Index: measuring the secondary impact of skin disease. *Br J Dermatol*. 2007;**156**:528-38.

[15] Boehncke WH, Schon MP. Psoriasis. *Lancet*. 2015;**386**:983-94.

[16] Frischknecht L, Vecellio M, Selmi C. The role of epigenetics and immunological imbalance in the etiopathogenesis of psoriasis and psoriatic arthritis. *Ther Adv Musculoskelet Dis*. 2019;**11**:1759720X19886505.

[17] Michalek IM, Loring B, John SM. A systematic review of worldwide epidemiology of psoriasis. *J Eur Acad Dermatol Venereol*. 2017;**31**:205-12.

[18] Parisi R, Symmons DP, Griffiths CE, Ashcroft DM, Identification, Management of P, et al. Global epidemiology of psoriasis: a systematic

review of incidence and prevalence. *J Invest Dermatol*. 2013;**133**:377-85.

[19] AlQassimi S, AlBrashdi S, Galadari H, Hashim MJ. Global burden of psoriasis - comparison of regional and global epidemiology, 1990 to 2017. *Int J Dermatol*. 2020;**59**:566-71.

[20] Mehrmal S, Uppal P, Nedley N, Giesey RL, Delost GR. The global, regional, and national burden of psoriasis in 195 countries and territories, 1990-2017: A systematic analysis from the Global Burden of Disease Study 2017. *J Am Acad Dermatol*. 2020.

[21] Griffiths CE, Barker JN. Pathogenesis and clinical features of psoriasis. *Lancet*. 2007;**370**:263-71.

[22] WHO. World Health Organization. EXECUTIVE BOARD. EB133/5. 133rd session. 5 April 2013. Provisional agenda item 6.2. Psoriasis. [WWW document] 2013. [cited 2020 May 13]. Available from: https://apps.who.int/gb/ebwha/pdf_files/EB133/B133_5-en.pdf. 2013.

[23] Arias-Santiago S, Orgaz-Molina J, Castellote-Caballero L, Arrabal-Polo MA, Garcia-Rodriguez S, Perandres-Lopez R, et al. Atheroma plaque, metabolic syndrome and inflammation in patients with psoriasis. *Eur J Dermatol*. 2012;**22**:337-44.

[24] Martinez-Lopez A, Blasco-Morente G, Giron-Prieto MS, Arrabal-Polo MA, Luque-Valenzuela M, Luna-Del Castillo JD, et al. Linking of psoriasis with osteopenia and osteoporosis: A cross-sectional study. *Indian J Dermatol Venereol Leprol*. 2019;**85**:153-9.

[25] Oliveira Mde F, Rocha Bde O, Duarte GV. Psoriasis: classical and emerging comorbidities. *An Bras Dermatol*. 2015;**90**:9-20.

[26] Orgaz-Molina J, Buendia-Eisman A, Arrabal-Polo MA, Ruiz JC, Arias-Santiago S. Deficiency of serum concentration of 25-hydroxyvitamin D in psoriatic patients: a case-control study. *J Am Acad Dermatol*. 2012;**67**:931-8.

[27] Abuabara K, Azfar RS, Shin DB, Neimann AL, Troxel AB, Gelfand JM. Cause-specific mortality in patients with severe psoriasis: a population-based cohort study in the U.K. *Br J Dermatol*. 2010;**163**:586-92.

[28] Lockshin B, Balagula Y, Merola JF. Interleukin 17, inflammation, and cardiovascular risk in patients with psoriasis. *J Am Acad Dermatol*. 2018;**79**:345-52.

[29] Nicholas MN, Gooderham M. Psoriasis, Depression, and Suicidality. *Skin Therapy Lett*. 2017;**22**:1-4.

[30] Molina-Leyva A, Salvador-Rodriguez L, Martinez-Lopez A, Ruiz-Carrascosa JC, Arias-Santiago S. Association Between Psoriasis and Sexual and Erectile Dysfunction in Epidemiologic Studies: A Systematic Review. *JAMA Dermatol*. 2019;**155**:98-106.

[31] Feldman SR, Burudpakdee C, Gala S, Nanavaty M, Mallya UG. The economic burden of psoriasis: a systematic literature review. *Expert Rev Pharmacoecon Outcomes Res*. 2014;**14**:685-705.

[32] Halioua B, Maccari F, Fougerousse AC, Parier J, Reguiai Z, Taieb C, et al. Impact of patient psoriasis on partner quality of life, sexuality and empathy feelings: a study in 183 couples. *J Eur Acad Dermatol Venereol*. 2020;**34**:2044-50.

[33] Stiff KM, Glines KR, Porter CL, Cline A, Feldman SR. Current pharmacological treatment guidelines for psoriasis and psoriatic arthritis. *Expert Rev Clin Pharmacol*. 2018;**11**: 1209-18.

[34] Menter A, Strober BE, Kaplan DH, Kivelevitch D, Prater EF, Stoff B, et al. Joint AAD-NPF guidelines of care for the management and treatment of psoriasis with biologics. *J Am Acad Dermatol*. 2019;**80**:1029-72.

[35] Jemec GB. Clinical practice. Hidradenitis suppurativa. *N Engl J Med*. 2012;**366**:158-64.

[36] Alikhan A, Lynch PJ, Eisen DB. Hidradenitis suppurativa: a comprehensive review. *J Am Acad Dermatol*. 2009;**60**:539-61.

[37] Revuz JE, Canoui-Poitrine F, Wolkenstein P, Viallette C, Gabison G, Pouget F, et al. Prevalence and factors associated with hidradenitis suppurativa: Results from two case-control studies. *Journal of the American Academy of Dermatology*. 2008;**59**: 596-601.

[38] Kirsten N, Petersen J, Hagenstrom K, Augustin M. Epidemiology of hidradenitis suppurativa in Germany - an observational cohort study based on a multisource approach. *J Eur Acad Dermatol*. 2020;**34**:174-9.

[39] Jemec GBE, Heidenheim M, Nielsen NH. The prevalence of hidradenitis suppurativa and its potential precursor lesions. *Journal of the American Academy of Dermatology*. 1996;**35**:191-4.

[40] Cosmatos I, Matcho A, Weinstein R, Montgomery MO, Stang P. Analysis of patient claims data to determine the prevalence of hidradenitis suppurativa in the United States. *Journal of the American Academy of Dermatology*. 2013;**68**:412-9.

[41] Nguyen TV, Damiani G, Orenstein LAV, Hamzavi I, Jemec GB. Hidradenitis suppurativa: an update on epidemiology, phenotypes, diagnosis, pathogenesis, comorbidities and quality of life. *J Eur Acad Dermatol Venereol*. 2020.

[42] Matusiak L. Profound consequences of hidradenitis suppurativa: a review. *Br J Dermatol*. 2018.

[43] Tzellos T, Zouboulis CC. Review of Comorbidities of Hidradenitis Suppurativa: Implications for Daily Clinical Practice. *Dermatol Ther (Heidelb)*. 2020;**10**:63-71.

[44] Machado MO, Stergiopoulos V, Maes M, Kurdyak PA, Lin PY, Wang LJ, et al. Depression and Anxiety in Adults With Hidradenitis Suppurativa: A Systematic Review and Meta-analysis. *JAMA Dermatol*. 2019.

[45] Jalenques I, Ciortianu L, Pereira B, D'Incan M, Lauron S, Rondepierre F. The prevalence and odds of anxiety and depression in children and adults with hidradenitis suppurativa: Systematic review and meta-analysis. *J Am Acad Dermatol*. 2020;**83**:542-53.

[46] Cuenca-Barrales C, Montero-Vilchez T, Szepietowski JC, Matusiak L, Molina-Leyva A. Sexual impairment in patients with hidradenitis suppurativa: a systematic review. *J Eur Acad Dermatol Venereol*. 2020.

[47] Cuenca-Barrales C, Molina-Leyva A. Sexuality in Patients with Hidradenitis Suppurativa: Beliefs, Behaviors and Needs. *Int J Environ Res Public Health*. 2020;**17**.

[48] Marvel J, Vlahiotis A, Sainski-Nguyen A, Willson T, Kimball A. Disease burden and cost of hidradenitis suppurativa: a retrospective examination of US administrative claims data. *BMJ Open*. 2019;**9**: e030579.

[49] Desai N, Shah P. High burden of hospital resource utilization in patients with hidradenitis suppurativa in England: a retrospective cohort study

using hospital episode statistics. *Br J Dermatol*. 2017;**176**:1048-55.

[50] Tzellos T, Yang H, Mu F, Calimlim B, Signorovitch J. Impact of hidradenitis suppurativa on work loss, indirect costs and income. *Br J Dermatol*. 2019;**181**:147-54.

[51] Wlodarek K, Glowaczewska A, Matusiak L, Szepietowski JC. Psychosocial burden of Hidradenitis Suppurativa patients' partners. *J Eur Acad Dermatol Venereol*. 2020;**34**:1822-7.

[52] Ramos-Alejos-Pita C, Arias-Santiago S, Molina-Leyva A. Quality of Life in Cohabitants of Patients with Hidradenitis Suppurativa: A Cross-sectional Study. *Int J Environ Res Public Health*. 2020;**17**.

[53] Marasca C, Napolitano M, Monfrecola G, Masara A, Annunziata MC, Donnarumma M, et al. Quality of life in people living with patients suffering from hidradenitis suppurativa. *J Eur Acad Dermatol Venereol*. 2020;**34**:e342-e3.

[54] Alikhan A, Sayed C, Alavi A, Alhusayen R, Brassard A, Burkhart C, et al. North American clinical management guidelines for hidradenitis suppurativa: A publication from the United States and Canadian Hidradenitis Suppurativa Foundations: Part II: Topical, intralesional, and systemic medical management. *J Am Acad Dermatol*. 2019;**81**:91-101.

[55] Zouboulis CC, Bechara FG, Dickinson-Blok JL, Gulliver W, Horvath B, Hughes R, et al. Hidradenitis suppurativa/acne inversa: a practical framework for treatment optimization - systematic review and recommendations from the HS ALLIANCE working group. *J Eur Acad Dermatol Venereol*. 2019;**33**:19-31.

[56] Gulliver W, Zouboulis CC, Prens E, Jemec GB, Tzellos T. Evidence-based approach to the treatment of hidradenitis suppurativa/acne inversa, based on the European guidelines for hidradenitis suppurativa. *Rev Endocr Metab Disord*. 2016;**17**:343-51.

[57] Kimball AB, Sobell JM, Zouboulis CC, Gu Y, Williams DA, Sundaram M, et al. HiSCR (Hidradenitis Suppurativa Clinical Response): a novel clinical endpoint to evaluate therapeutic outcomes in patients with hidradenitis suppurativa from the placebo-controlled portion of a phase 2 adalimumab study. *J Eur Acad Dermatol Venereol*. 2016;**30**:989-94.

[58] Montero-Vilchez T, Salvador-Rodriguez L, Sanchez-Diaz M, Cuenca-Barrales C, Martinez-Lopez A, Arias-Santiago S, et al. Clinical selection criteria in new clinical trials of hidradenitis suppurativa: External validity and implications on the daily clinical practice. *Dermatol Ther*. 2020:e14254.

[59] Tappenden P, Carroll C, Stevens JW, Rawdin A, Grimm S, Clowes M, et al. Adalimumab for Treating Moderate-to-Severe Hidradenitis Suppurativa: An Evidence Review Group Perspective of a NICE Single Technology Appraisal. *Pharmacoeconomics*. 2017;**35**:805-15.

[60] Willems D, Charokopou M, Evers S, Hiligsmann M. Early health economic modelling for a treatment candidate in hidradenitis suppurativa. *J Med Econ*. 2020:1-9.

[61] Williams HC, Dellavalle RP, Garner *S. Acne* vulgaris. *Lancet*. 2012;**379**:361-72.

[62] Tan JK, Bhate K. A global perspective on the epidemiology of acne. *Br J Dermatol*. 2015;**172 Suppl 1**:3-12.

[63] Moradi Tuchayi S, Makrantonaki E, Ganceviciene R, Dessinioti C, Feldman SR, Zouboulis CC. Acne

vulgaris. *Nat Rev Dis Primers*. 2015;**1**:15029.

[64] Claudel JP, Auffret N, Leccia MT, Poli F, Dreno B. Acne and nutrition: hypotheses, myths and facts. *J Eur Acad Dermatol Venereol*. 2018;**32**:1631-7.

[65] Sood S, Jafferany M, Vinaya Kumar S. Depression, psychiatric comorbidities, and psychosocial implications associated with acne vulgaris. *J Cosmet Dermatol*. 2020;**19**:3177-82.

[66] Altunay IK, Ozkur E, Dalgard FJ, Gieler U, Tomas Aragones L, Lien L, et al. Psychosocial Aspects of Adult Acne: Data from 13 European Countries. *Acta Derm Venereol*. 2020;**100**:adv00051.

[67] Bez Y, Yesilova Y, Kaya MC, Sir A. High social phobia frequency and related disability in patients with acne vulgaris. *Eur J Dermatol*. 2011;**21**:756-60.

[68] Martinez-Garcia E, Arias-Santiago S, Herrera-Acosta E, Affleck A, Herrera-Ceballos E, Buendia-Eisman A. Quality of Life of Cohabitants of People Living with Acne. *Acta Derm Venereol*. 2020;**100**:adv00290.

[69] Zaenglein AL, Pathy AL, Schlosser BJ, Alikhan A, Baldwin HE, Berson DS, et al. Guidelines of care for the management of acne vulgaris. *J Am Acad Dermatol*. 2016;**74**:945-73 e33.

[70] Simpson N. Effect of isotretinoin on the quality of life of patients with acne. *Pharmacoeconomics*. 1994;**6**:108-13.

[71] Davis SA, Himmler S, Feldman SR. Cost-effectiveness analysis of using dermatologists versus pediatricians to treat mild to moderate acne. *Dermatol Online J*. 2017;**23**.

[72] Silverberg JI. Public Health Burden and Epidemiology of Atopic Dermatitis. Dermatol Clin. 2017;35(3):283-289. doi:10.1016/j.det.2017.02.002

[73] Weidinger S, Novak N. Atopic dermatitis. Lancet (London, England). 2016;387(10023):1109-1122. doi:10.1016/S0140-6736(15)00149-X

[74] Brunner PM, Leung DYM, Guttman-Yassky E. Immunologic, microbial, and epithelial interactions in atopic dermatitis. Ann allergy, asthma Immunol Off Publ Am Coll Allergy, Asthma, Immunol. 2018;120(1):34-41. doi:10.1016/j.anai.2017.09.055

[75] Kim J, Kim BE, Leung DYM. Pathophysiology of atopic dermatitis: Clinical implications. Allergy asthma Proc. 2019;40(2):84-92. doi:10.2500/aap.2019.40.4202

[76] Liang Y, Chang C, Lu Q. The Genetics and Epigenetics of Atopic Dermatitis-Filaggrin and Other Polymorphisms. Clin Rev Allergy Immunol. 2016;51(3):315-328. doi:10.1007/s12016-015-8508-5

[77] Loukogeorgakis SP, De Coppi P. Stem cells from amniotic fluid--Potential for regenerative medicine. Best Pract Res Clin Obstet Gynaecol. 2016;31:45-57. doi:10.1016/j.bpobgyn.2015.08.009

[78] Renert-Yuval Y, Guttman-Yassky E. New treatments for atopic dermatitis targeting beyond IL-4/IL-13 cytokines. Ann allergy, asthma Immunol Off Publ Am Coll Allergy, Asthma, Immunol. 2020;124(1):28-35. doi:10.1016/j.anai.2019.10.005

[79] Silverberg JI. Comorbidities and the impact of atopic dermatitis. Ann allergy, asthma Immunol Off Publ Am Coll Allergy, Asthma, Immunol. 2019;123(2):144-151. doi:10.1016/j.anai.2019.04.020

[80] González-Cervera J, Arias Á, Redondo-González O, Cano-Mollinedo MM, Terreehorst I, Lucendo AJ. Association between atopic manifestations and eosinophilic

esophagitis: A systematic review and meta-analysis. Ann allergy, asthma Immunol Off Publ Am Coll Allergy, Asthma, Immunol. 2017;118(5):582-590.e2. doi:10.1016/j.anai.2017.02.006

[81] Hamann CR, Hamann D, Egeberg A, Johansen JD, Silverberg J, Thyssen JP. Association between atopic dermatitis and contact sensitization: A systematic review and meta-analysis. J Am Acad Dermatol. 2017;77(1):70-78. doi:https://doi.org/10.1016/j.jaad.2017.02.001

[82] Ascott A, Mulick A, Yu AM, et al. Atopic eczema and major cardiovascular outcomes: A systematic review and meta-analysis of population-based studies. J Allergy Clin Immunol. 2019;143(5):1821-1829. doi:10.1016/j.jaci.2018.11.030

[83] Totté JEE, van der Feltz WT, Hennekam M, van Belkum A, van Zuuren EJ, Pasmans SGMA. Prevalence and odds of *Staphylococcus aureus* carriage in atopic dermatitis: a systematic review and meta-analysis. Br J Dermatol. 2016;175(4):687-695. doi:10.1111/bjd.14566

[84] Serrano L, Patel KR, Silverberg JI. Association between atopic dermatitis and extracutaneous bacterial and mycobacterial infections: A systematic review and meta-analysis. J Am Acad Dermatol. 2019;80(4):904-912. doi:10.1016/j.jaad.2018.11.028

[85] Fishbein AB, Silverberg JI, Wilson EJ, Ong PY. Update on Atopic Dermatitis: Diagnosis, Severity Assessment, and Treatment Selection. J allergy Clin Immunol Pract. 2020;8(1):91-101. doi:10.1016/j.jaip.2019.06.044

[86] Silverberg JI, Gelfand JM, Margolis DJ, et al. Patient burden and quality of life in atopic dermatitis in US adults: A population-based cross-sectional study. Ann Allergy, Asthma Immunol. 2018;121(3):340-347. doi:https://doi.org/10.1016/j.anai.2018.07.006

[87] Xu X, van Galen LS, Koh MJA, et al. Factors influencing quality of life in children with atopic dermatitis and their caregivers: a cross-sectional study. Sci Rep. 2019;9(1):15990. doi:10.1038/s41598-019-51129-5

[88] Chernyshov P V. Health-related quality of life in adult atopic dermatitis and psoriatic patients matched by disease severity. G Ital di dermatologia e Venereol organo Uff Soc Ital di dermatologia e Sifilogr. 2016;151(1):37-43.

[89] Patel KR, Singam V, Vakharia PP, et al. Measurement properties of three assessments of burden used in atopic dermatitis in adults. Br J Dermatol. 2019;180(5):1083-1089. doi:10.1111/bjd.17243

[90] Ezzedine K, Shourick J, Merhand S, Sampogna F, Taïeb C. Impact of Atopic Dermatitis in Adolescents and their Parents: A French Study. Acta Derm Venereol. 2020;100(17):adv00294. doi:10.2340/00015555-3653

[91] Gieler U, Schoof S, Gieler T, Scheewe S, Schut C, Kupfer J. Atopic Eczema and Stress among Single Parents and Families: An Empirical Study of 96 Mothers. Acta Derm Venereol. 2017;97(1):42-46. doi:10.2340/00015555-2457

[92] Jang HJ, Hwang S, Ahn Y, Lim DH, Sohn M, Kim JH. Family quality of life among families of children with atopic dermatitis. Asia Pac Allergy. 2016;6(4):213-219. doi:10.5415/apallergy.2016.6.4.213

[93] Han JW, Lee H. Actor and partner effects of parenting stress and co-parenting on marital conflict among parents of children with atopic dermatitis. BMC Pediatr.

2020;20(1):141. doi:10.1186/s12887-020-02035-7

[94] Misery L, Seneschal J, Reguiai Z, et al. The impact of atopic dermatitis on sexual health. J Eur Acad Dermatol Venereol. 2019;33(2):428-432. doi:10.1111/jdv.15223

[95] Ludwig CM, Fernandez JM, Hsiao JL, Shi VY. The Interplay of Atopic Dermatitis and Sexual Health. Dermat contact, atopic, Occup drug. 2020;31(5):303-308. doi:10.1097/DER.0000000000000617

[96] Silverberg JI, Gelfand JM, Margolis DJ, et al. Health Utility Scores of Atopic Dermatitis in US Adults. J Allergy Clin Immunol Pract. 2019;7(4):1246-1252.e1. doi:https://doi.org/10.1016/j.jaip.2018.11.043

[97] Chylla R, Schnopp C, Volz T. Basic skin care in atopic dermatitis - new and established treatment options. J der Dtsch Dermatologischen Gesellschaft = J Ger Soc Dermatology JDDG. 2018;16(8):976-979. doi:10.1111/ddg.13594

[98] Chun PIF, Lehman H. Current and Future Monoclonal Antibodies in the Treatment of Atopic Dermatitis. Clin Rev Allergy Immunol. 2020;59(2):208-219. doi:10.1007/s12016-020-08802-9

[99] Drucker AM, Wang AR, Li W-Q, Sevetson E, Block JK, Qureshi AA. The Burden of Atopic Dermatitis: Summary of a Report for the National Eczema Association. J Invest Dermatol. 2017;137(1):26-30. doi:10.1016/j.jid.2016.07.012

[100] Zimmermann M, Rind D, Chapman R, Kumar V, Kahn S, Carlson J. Economic Evaluation of Dupilumab for Moderate-to-Severe Atopic Dermatitis: A Cost-Utility Analysis. J Drugs Dermatol. 2018;17(7):750-756.

[101] Lolli F, Pallotti F, Rossi A, et al. Androgenetic alopecia: a review. Endocrine. 2017;57(1):9-17. doi:10.1007/s12020-017-1280-y

[102] Severi G, Sinclair R, Hopper JL, et al. Androgenetic alopecia in men aged 40-69 years: prevalence and risk factors. Br J Dermatol. 2003;149(6):1207-1213. doi:10.1111/j.1365-2133.2003.05565.x

[103] Gan DCC, Sinclair RD. Prevalence of male and female pattern hair loss in Maryborough. J Investig dermatology Symp Proc. 2005;10(3):184-189. doi:10.1111/j.1087-0024.2005.10102.x

[104] Kim B-K, Choe SJ, Chung H-C, Oh S-S, Lee W-S. Gender-specific risk factors for androgenetic alopecia in the Korean general population: Associations with medical comorbidities and general health behaviors. Int J Dermatol. 2018;57(2):183-192. doi:10.1111/ijd.13843

[105] Gonul M, Cemil BC, Ayvaz HH, Cankurtaran E, Ergin C, Gurel MS. Comparison of quality of life in patients with androgenetic alopecia and alopecia areata. An Bras Dermatol. 2018;93(5):651-658. doi:10.1590/abd1806-4841.20186131

[106] Gupta S, Goyal I, Mahendra A. Quality of Life Assessment in Patients with Androgenetic Alopecia. Int J Trichology. 2019;11(4):147-152. doi:10.4103/ijt.ijt_6_19

[107] Ghimire RB. Impact on Quality of Life in Patients who came with Androgenetic Alopecia for Hair Transplantion Surgery in a Clinic. JNMA J Nepal Med Assoc. 2018;56(212):763-765.

[108] Sancak EB, Oguz S, Akbulut T, Uludag A, Akbas A, Kurt O, Akbulut MF. Female sexual dysfunction in androgenetic alopecia: Case-control study. Can Urol Assoc J. 2016

Jul-Aug;10(7-8):E251-E256. doi: 10.5489/cuaj.3582.

[109] Rossi A, Anzalone A, Fortuna MC, et al. Multi-therapies in androgenetic alopecia: review and clinical experiences. Dermatol Ther. 2016;29(6):424-432. doi:10.1111/dth.12390

[110] Campese VM. Minoxidil: a review of its pharmacological properties and therapeutic use. Drugs. 1981;22(4): 257-278. doi:10.2165/0000 3495-198122040-00001

[111] Randolph M, Tosti A. Oral minoxidil treatment for hair loss: A review of efficacy and safety. J Am Acad Dermatol. 2020;Jul 1(S0190-9622(20)32109-5). doi:10.1016/j.jaad.2020.06.1009

[112] Villasante Fricke AC, Miteva M. Epidemiology and burden of alopecia areata: a systematic review. Clin Cosmet Investig Dermatol. 2015;8:397-403. doi:10.2147/CCID.S53985

[113] Strazzulla LC, Wang EHC, Avila L, et al. Alopecia areata: Disease characteristics, clinical evaluation, and new perspectives on pathogenesis. J Am Acad Dermatol. 2018;78(1):1-12. doi:10.1016/j.jaad.2017.04.1141

[114] Han TY, Lee JH, Noh TK, et al. Alopecia areata and overt thyroid diseases: A nationwide population-based study. J Dermatol. 2018;45(12):1411-1417. doi:10.1111/1346-8138.14648

[115] Huang KP, Mullangi S, Guo Y, Qureshi AA. Autoimmune, atopic, and mental health comorbid conditions associated with alopecia areata in the United States. JAMA dermatology. 2013;149(7):789-794. doi:10.1001/jamadermatol.2013.3049

[116] Lee S, Lee H, Lee CH, Lee W-S. Comorbidities in alopecia areata: A systematic review and meta-analysis. J Am Acad Dermatol. 2019;80(2):466-477.e16. doi:10.1016/j.jaad.2018.07.013

[117] Ruiz-Doblado S, Carrizosa A, García-Hernández MJ. Alopecia areata: psychiatric comorbidity and adjustment to illness. Int J Dermatol. 2003;42(6): 434-437. doi:10.1046/j.1365-4362.2003.01340.x

[118] Colón EA, Popkin MK, Callies AL, Dessert NJ, Hordinsky MK. Lifetime prevalence of psychiatric disorders in patients with alopecia areata. Compr Psychiatry. 1991;32(3):245-251. doi:10.1016/0010-440x(91)90045-e

[119] Sellami R, Masmoudi J, Ouali U, et al. The relationship between alopecia areata and alexithymia, anxiety and depression: a case-control study. Indian J Dermatol. 2014;59(4):421. doi:10.4103/0019-5154.135525

[120] Toussi A, Barton VR, Le ST, Agbai ON, Kiuru M. Psychosocial and psychiatric comorbidities and health-related quality of life in alopecia areata: a systematic review. J Am Acad Dermatol. June 2020. doi:10.1016/j.jaad.2020.06.047

[121] Vélez-Muñiz RDC, Peralta-Pedrero ML, Jurado-Santa Cruz F, Morales-Sánchez MA. Psychological Profile and Quality of Life of Patients with Alopecia Areata. Ski appendage Disord. 2019;5(5):293-298. doi:10.1159/000497166

[122] Rencz F, Gulácsi L, Péntek M, Wikonkál N, Baji P, Brodszky V. Alopecia areata and health-related quality of life: a systematic review and meta-analysis. Br J Dermatol. 2016;175(3):561-571. doi:10.1111/bjd.14497

[123] Li SJ, Huang KP, Joyce C, Mostaghimi A. The Impact of Alopecia Areata on Sexual Quality of Life. Int J Trichology. 2018 Nov-Dec;10(6): 271-274. doi: 10.4103/ijt.ijt_93_18. PMID: 30783334; PMCID: PMC6369646.

[124] Arias Santiago S, Montero-Vílchez T, López-Nevot García MA, Torres Aroza M, Rodríguez Tejero A, Buendía-Eisman A. Análisis de la calidad de vida en convivientes de pacientes con alopecia areata y frontal fibrosante. Poster presented at Virtual Congress AEDV Autumn; 2020 Nov 19-21; Spain.

[125] Rossi A, Muscianese M, Piraccini BM, et al. Italian Guidelines in diagnosis and treatment of alopecia areata. G Ital di dermatologia e Venereol organo Uff Soc Ital di dermatologia e Sifilogr. 2019;154(6):609-623. doi:10.23736/S0392-0488.19.06458-7

[126] Strazzulla LC, Wang EHC, Avila L, et al. Alopecia areata: An appraisal of new treatment approaches and overview of current therapies. J Am Acad Dermatol. 2018;78(1):15-24. doi:10.1016/j.jaad.2017.04.1142

[127] Saceda-Corralo D, Pindado-Ortega C, Moreno-Arrones ÓM, et al. Health-Related Quality of Life in Patients With Frontal Fibrosing Alopecia. JAMA dermatology. 2018;154(4):479-480. doi:10.1001/jamadermatol.2017.6330

Chapter 6

Psychological Intervention Based on Psychoneuroimmunology in Children and Adults

Margarita del Valle Chacin Fuenmayor and Josymar Chacin de Fernandez

Abstract

Psychoneuroimmunology (PNI) is a field that has developed significantly during the last three decades; it has come to scientifically demonstrate the importance of the mind in the prevention, development and treatment of diseases. Throughout this chapter, we describe the evolution of PNI, the interaction of these systems to actively develop them, not only in adults but also in children. Similarly, it explains the influence of stress on the health of the individual and the importance of knowledge of psychoneuroimmunology to achieve the proper management of disease and quality of life. It also accounts for how psychological interventions have been proven effective and can serve as a model for researching and treating other diseases.

Keywords: psychoneuroimmunology (PNI), stress, psychological intervention, children, quality of life

1. Introduction

This chapter will describe the main clinical implications of psychoneuroimmunology and how to improve clinical evolution, quality of life and immunity of adults and children. The investigation of the multiple relationships between emotions and human cognition and health is an area of study that involves much knowledge, such as neurosciences, endocrinology, immunology, pharmacology, psychology, and psychiatry. These knowledge areas provide a partial vision to make a complete approach to the relationship between the disease, the body and the mind-brain.

The concept of health is a complex process, and it is based on a balance between biological, social and psychological factors. Engel, in 1977 [1], worked on the recognition of the intricate relationship between disease, body and mind-brain, argued that biological factors, as well as genetic factors, are not enough to explain all the phenomena that have to do with health, and that if you want to understand the origin and evolution of the disease, you must take into account the interaction of psychological and social factors in addition to genetic and biological factors; He also emphasized his criticism of the traditional biomedical model that tends to separate the mind-brain and the body; model where the body is conceived as a machine that must be repaired, leaving aside the emotions; patients are seen almost as objects, and their subjective perception is not relevant in medical evaluation and management, contributing to the dehumanized procedure of traditional medicine.

Considering the relevance around the advances in the medical field, this chapter will provide a better understanding of Psychoneuroimmunology and describe the psychological protocols developed for adult and children, which has been proven to improve clinical evolution, quality of life and immunity.

2. Psychoneuroimmunology (PNI)

Psychoneuroimmunology (PNI) consolidates itself as an interdisciplinary research field towards the end of the 70s. It owes its name to the psychologist Robert Ader, who first introduced the term in his presidential address of the American psychosomatic society in 1980 [2]. Later this neologism was presented more formally by Ader, 1981 as the title of a landmark book of this novel discipline in which state of the art was presented, emphasizing the central nervous system's role in the interaction of behavior and the immune system [3].

One of the newest research fields resulting from the biopsychosocial conception of health is psychoneuroimmunology (PNI), which embraces the main guideline of this model, such as the analysis of the interaction between psychosocial and biological factors in etiology, evolution and treatment of the disease. Psychoneuroimmunology is a prominent new scientific field where many sciences converge responsible for the study, analysis, understanding, and application of the complex interactions between behavior and the three systems that guarantee the human body's homeostasis, between the nervous system, the endocrine and immune system [4].

This hybrid new discipline tries to demonstrate if the mind-brain mediates the susceptibility to illness or intervenes to recover a physical ailment, an infectious or autoimmune disease. The relationship of some psychological processes with alterations of the immune system and the interrelation of mental illnesses, mainly emotional and affective, with impaired immune function [5]. Psychoneuroimmunology provides more detailed knowledge of the intricate biological dynamics of human health. It provides novel complementary medical options or techniques and invites exploring alternative non-linear models to address the health-disease process. PNI is thus a discipline that establishes a meeting point for the different traditional health fields [2].

PNI is thus a discipline that establishes a meeting point for the different traditional health fields. Many research pieces have proven the relevance to the scientific field, which has helped to acknowledge and understand these systems' link to improve adults and children's health integrally.

3. Stress and psychoneuroimmunology

Studies on the effect of stress on the immune system have allowed understanding the complex interaction between the nervous, endocrine and immune systems, which has allowed that in situations of stress, the human organism has protection mechanisms to preserve homeostasis.

In the fourteenth century, the term stress began to refer to difficult, adverse, suffering and negative situations. However, it was not until 1857, when Claude Bernard stated that environmental changes could alter the body. In 1929 the neurologist Walter Cannon recognized that stressors that cause physiological reactions resulting from threatening or adverse situations could be physical and/or emotional. Cannon also warned, later in 1932, about the importance of the person maintaining an internal balance that he called homeostasis and that in case of intense changes, a readjustment occurred through the endocrine and vegetative system [6].

Later, Hans Seyle, physiologist and physician, considered by many to be the father of the modern concept of stress, defined it in 1936 in the British journal Nature the General Adaptation Syndrome (SGA), also known as Seyle's Law, as an automatic mechanism that is triggered by any stressful situation and that involves a set of reactions that mobilize energy reserves that implies activation of the hypothalamic-hypophysical-adrenal axis and the central nervous system, which makes the body go through three phases: alarm, resistance or adaptation of the organism and exhaustion, being able, if the threat is sufficiently severe and prolonged, even cause death [6].

When stress exceeds certain limits, the immune system is affected, numerous organs of our body, and there is a propensity for the appearance or aggravation of diseases by weakening certain immune cells that make people more susceptible to the pathogens that cause infections such as asthma, rheumatoid arthritis, herpes simplex, tuberculosis, cancer and the progression of HIV to AIDS, among others [6].

Among the consequences of chronic stress on the immune, central nervous and endocrine systems, Ortega Navas, M, 2011, highlights the following:

Chronic stress effects on health	
Immune system	• Depressed immune activity. • Weakening of the immune system: Acceleration of infectious processes, colds and autoimmune diseases. • Problems with blood clotting. • Reactivation of inflammatory diseases: atopic dermatitis and psoriasis. • Increased retention of the virus in tissues
Nervous system	• Depression, anxiety, loss of sleep. • Cognitive abilities such as memory and the ability to take decisions can be adversely affected. • Increased risk of developing neurodegenerative diseases such as multiple sclerosis, central nervous system infections, and others inflammatory diseases.
Endocrine System	• Increase of sugars and fats in the blood. • Hypothyroidism and hyperthyroidism. • Cushing's syndrome. • Hormonal changes: increased secretion of catecholamines and cortisol, which have an immunosuppressive effect. • Modification of prolactin, growth hormone and ß-endorphin levels

On the other hand, stress is also necessary and positive in our lives' evolution at certain levels since it constitutes an essential part. Positive stress is a means of adaptation to daily situations, a means for productivity, creativity, increases alertness, improves concentration, and decision-making, making us feel safe and better prepared to face and definitively find ourselves in a more balanced situation the face of adversity and disease.

Sometimes we adults have the fantasy that children are not stressed because we see them playing or entertaining themselves in their activities, which is absolutely false since, on the contrary, the fact that the child has a high power to imagine also causes you to present abundant thoughts and that when events are not clearly explained or because of your cognitive level, you cannot interpret them clearly, it is possible that the thoughts are negative, which generates high stress and therefore also affects your immune system.

In this sense, it is essential to provide children with information, according to their age, of the events that are being generated, whether they are associated with themselves, as in the case of their health, as if it is about the people around you. It is recommended to address critical situations such as divorces, moves, bereavement and maintain close contact, with the openness to answer any question that arises at the time, to reduce the anxiety of uncertainty that is very harmful to the child.

4. Emotions and psychoneuroimmunology

Emotions govern all the organism's systems. The field of psychoneuroimmunology is studying how emotions are translated into chemical substances (information molecules) that can trigger chain reactions that affect internal chemistry, optimizing or weakening our functional state. Furthermore, that impacts our immune system, endocrine system, nervous system and other systems of our body. In fact, if we repress the expression of emotions, we also repress our organic functions, which in the long term translates into discomfort or diseases [6].

Research indicates that positive emotions can be enhanced and help prevent certain diseases' appearance. What we do and what we think has positive and negative effects on our physical and emotional health. Positive emotions allow us, in addition to supporting the difficulties of an illness and facilitating its recovery by triggering a series of positive effects on our metabolism that strengthen our health, achieve, among other goals, healthy self-esteem, satisfaction for the work well done and making more effective decisions and ultimately, improve our quality of life. In fact, positive emotions also help make people more resistant to adversity and help build psychological resilience [7].

Maruso in 2009 [8], considered that emotions influence immunity and that the third revolution in medicine is precisely psychoneuroimmunoendocrinology. He insists that the mind and the body are intrinsically linked and that as a result of the mind–body interaction, reactions are triggered that affect internal chemistry, optimizing or weakening our functional state and that it is in our own hands to launch a new culture of health which implies that people are capable of maintaining and ensuring health on a physical and mental level.

Advances in psychoneuroimmunology indicate that emotional states can modify and alter health in general so that positive emotions help the person be better able to overcome diseases that may arise in life. Likewise, Ortega Navas in 2009, affirms that emotions play a vital role in health, "they are an undeniable part of our lives and are fundamental for its positive state by helping to promote healthy behaviour; on the contrary, if they are negative, they are a risk to our health, they can constitute an activating or inhibiting signal of health symptoms or a disease".

The emotional attitude directly relates to the immune system, harmonizing better with good health than a negative attitude. A person who normally expresses happiness, good humor, love, friendship, joy and positivism is much less likely to contract a serious illness than another who, on the contrary, is angry, fearful, angry, depressed or apprehensive. In fact, when states of mind such as anger, fear, or hopelessness seize us, cortisol levels rise, which hinders the immune system's functioning.

In sum, although emotions play a decisive role in the onset and/or course of numerous diseases, among cardiovascular, respiratory, gastrointestinal, endocrine, muscular, dermatological disorders and alterations of the immune system stand out, it is important to highlight that emotional education as a subject. The current debate is increasingly being debated in educational settings, a consequence of the need to educate people to know themselves and others better to face the challenges of their daily work better and adopt healthier lifestyles. Its purpose is to help people prevent and reduce risk behaviors through skills training or avoid possible consequences.

5. Quality of life (QoL)

In recent times, the use of the term quality of life (QoL) has become frequent in a wide variety of contexts. Environmentalists emphasize the physical/biological environment, economists on parameters such as gross national product, doctors on symptoms, psychologists on human needs, and satisfaction. It follows that quality of life should be considered a multidisciplinary entity that is applicable and inherent to all society and the world, and its consideration by all leaders and scientists of humanity should be contemplated [9]. That is why it affirms Grau, in 1996 that the Quality-of-Life study invites us to abandon traditional positions and glimpse common sources of approach.

Almost all the authors agree that the term appears in the decade of Within Health Psychology; according to Grau, 1996, there are three large groups of problems when approaching the development of studies in Quality of Life. The first is that of its conceptual indistinctness, determined by its complex nature, the second referring to problems related to Quality of Life and the third problem inherent to the difficulties in its evaluation.

In pediatric literature, quality of life is defined as multidimensional. It includes the child's social, physical and emotional functioning and, if necessary, of his family [10]. Quality of life questionnaires have generally been validated related to health in which information from people close to children has been used; the ability of children to report their health status has not been considered adequate [11].

For a child, it is difficult to discriminate what is quality of life, since it has no source of comparison because due to its short life and the experiences it has had, it can build its concept of life, that is why on many scales to measure the quality of life of the child takes into account the perception that family members have of well-being in the child.

In this sense, a child's quality of life must be focused on providing a healthy environment, where they can fully develop their mental, physical and social capacities, allowing them to carry out childhood activities, reinforcing healthy beliefs that imply responsibility in their immunological condition.

5.1 Quality of life factors to consider in psychoneuroimmunology

Quality of Life is based on the construction that a person makes of their living standards according to their personal beliefs and environment, which determines their general well-being. Among the elements to consider are the following:

- Physical condition: In this aspect, the person's body conditions, energy level, vitality and the care that the person performs to maintain it, such as exercise and daily activity, are considered.

- Lifestyle and well-being: The way the person organizes their time in a balanced way, taking into personal account spaces, free time, interpersonal relationships, academic and work activities, indicates a healthy lifestyle.

- Healthy interpersonal relationships: The way the person relates is closely linked to personal well-being, especially close relationships.

- Physical and emotional symptoms: The awareness on the part of the person of the feelings he is experiencing at the physical and mental level is vital to assess her quality of life. In this regard, it is essential to consider the manifestations of pain in the organic and emotional sphere.

- Cognitive considerations: The mental construction that the person makes of his experience, that is, the perception of it, will influence how he responds to the environment and therefore affects his quality of life.

- Introspection, self-esteem and self-care: Intrapersonal communication, which implies communication with me, being compassionate and with a motivating dialog that reinforces self-esteem, is vital. Also accompanied by self-love that implies effective self-care in all areas.

- Sleep quality: it is considered relevant to validate problems falling asleep, interrupted sleep, insomnia, among others.

- Image and Sexuality: Self-image, added to the interest in sexual relations, desire and level of satisfaction, are factors to consider.

6. Psychological interventions based on psychoneuroimmunology in adults

Psychological interventions based on psychoneuroimmunology must be structured, taking into account:

1. Conviction in the patient of the mind–body relationship.

2. Knowledge of the immune system's primary authors and how it is related to the endocrine system and the nervous system.

3. Awareness in the patient that his mental and physical condition is linked to internal factors.

4. Identification of harmful behavioral patterns that must be modified to improve the quality of life.

6.1 Some techniques used in psychoneuroimmunology

6.1.1 Cognitive-behavioral psychotherapy

In this therapy applied to psychoneuroimmunology, the way of thinking on the immune response is explained to the person. A variety of cognitive strategies have helped identify the unhealthy beliefs that affect the individual's health condition. In general, the following process is followed:

- Identify the unhealthy belief

- Recognize the connections between thought - emotion - behavior.

- Examine the evidence that is for or against your thoughts.

- Correct distorted thoughts
- Replace cognitions with healthy beliefs.

6.1.2 Relaxation techniques

Relaxation techniques commonly used in psychoneuroimmunology usually include muscle relaxation and deep breathing to decrease neurovegetative activation. The training is the same as those used in clinical contexts, only adapting the procedure to health conditions.

6.1.3 Guided imagery techniques

The body does not discriminate between what we imagine and the actual events, which is why people who carry out a treatment based on psychoneuroimmunology must become aware of the power of their mind, and the care they must have at the time to worry in advance or imagine catastrophic events that alter their physical conditions.

Guided imagination in PNI includes 2 phases. Initially, the patient is guided through a relaxation process, and then he is induced to imagine the activation of his nervous, endocrine and immune systems to regulate his disease. This imagination can be general or specific according to his illness.

6.1.4 Psychoeducation

- Information about the disease:

In PNI, the patient must know all the details related to his disease. For example, if he has a tumor in any part of the body, it is essential that he can see the exams, know where it is located, its size, shape, texture, everything that allows him to imagine it or even draw it later.

- Treatment information:

In psychoneuroimmunology, the patient has an active role in his clinical condition and recovery of health; that is why he must know all the treatment details, the approximate time that he will receive them and the side effects. It is relevant that the patient can mentally potentiate or reject these treatments; that is why it is necessary to verify the distracted or catastrophic thoughts that can alter him emotionally and affect the immune response.

In children, it is very important to foster a collaborative attitude towards treatment, which stems from the understanding that some treatments, although painful, are promoting their health. Also, strengthening communication with their parents and health professionals.

- Information on the Immune System

The patient is required to recognize the main authors of the immune system to develop greater control over his physical symptoms and disease.

The content provided implies understanding the defense system, represented by white blood cells, and its function is to defend the person from viruses, bacteria, and any invading agent, such as tumor cells.

In psychoeducation, the different types of cells must be present, and their characteristics and general functions are explained according to the age group and cognitive level. Among the actors that stand out are T Lymphocyte, B Lymphocyte, Macrophage, Natural Killer Cell or NK and Neutrophil Polymorphonuclear.

7. Psychoneuroimmunology research in adults

There are several reasons to investigate whether a psychological intervention, in patients or healthy subjects, alters immunity: 1) Because it is possible to know if there is a causal relationship between psychological factors and the functioning of the immune system 2) because the improvement of the immunity obtained after the psychological intervention would be an added benefit (eg. Some stressors can cause a decrease in some forms of immunity. The psychological intervention would reduce stress and increase the multidisciplinary treatment of patients affected by organic diseases [5].

In this sense, any psychological variable can influence the appearance or the course and outcome of a certain disease in which the immune system is involved. As the psychological determinants that influence behavior can come directly from the CNS or indirectly through the stress response (hormonal mechanisms), any change in behavior that is associated with personality characteristics or coping styles in emergencies (stressful), as well as negative emotional states, could affect the immune system (for example, people who smoke or overeat when stressed or people who generate more stress than necessary in everyday situations by evaluating them exaggeratedly threatening). It also happens that, on some occasions, individuals see a threat where there is none (or they exaggerate it), resulting in the acquisition of a phobia; either they do not have adequate coping resources at a given moment (they do not know how to solve problems), or they have wrong ideas about how the world should work (irrational ideas or cognitive distortions) [10].

This can be evidence in a in work carried out by Antoni in 2003 [12], through a 10-week group program based on cognitive stress control and relaxation strategies, the results show that there are effects of psychological intervention on mood, as well as neuroendocrine changes in the HHC, HHG (Hypothalamic–Pituitary–Gonadal) axis as well as in the hormones of the Sympathetic Nervous System and the state of the Immune System in people infected with HIV. The changes produced by the effects of relaxation and cognitive coping strategies, and social support can mediate mood changes. In turn, these changes affect the regulation of adrenal hormones evaluated through changes in urinary cortisol, norepinephrine, and testosterone levels. As suggested by Antoni, the changes in these hormones as a result of the intervention could also explain, in part, the short-term changes in IgG antibodies and the longer-term changes in CD4 lymphocytes.

Similarly, Robinson in 2002 [13] showed encouraging results with an 8-week program to reduce stress in people infected with HIV. Subjects who received this treatment showed increased activity in the killer (NK) cells and their number. The same measurements were taken three months after completing the intervention, noting that the increases in NK cells and decreases in tension, anger or depression also remained, thus showing the subjects a much-improved state of mind.

In any case, the psychological influence of the mind on the body, and more specifically in the field of PNI since the mid-70s, have been treated from multidisciplinary approaches that include medicine, psychology, sociology, social work and even religion [3].

For this reason, and as far as psychologists are concerned, psychotherapies are usually directed towards two final objectives: to reduce or eliminate levels of stress and/or depression. Although stressors can be physical or psychological, the disparity between them is a mere illusion when it comes to the emission of a stress response [3]. Therefore, any treatment aimed at eliminating or reducing the stress response will be favoring the improvement of depression, this being, in this way, considered a dependent variable.

How an individual interprets and responds to a certain stressor determines its reaction (flight, freeze or flight) and the immune system's response and disease behaviors [14]. Therefore, any intervention from health psychology, designed to modulate stress, provides problem-solving strategies, identifies both phobic stimuli and real or potentially dangerous stimuli, adopts healthy behaviors, and interprets life events from a perspective adaptive (not a perfectionist or tremendous), will walk in the direction sought.

It has been scientifically proven that there are significant decreases in hormones related to stress, such as thyroxine or GH, decreases in Cortisol, THS, and prolactin have also been described during relaxation. Visualization produces increases in IgA levels in saliva. Decreases in the sensitivity of beta-adrenergic receptors measured in circulating lymphocytes have also been described without variations in the number of receptors or catecholamines' plasma concentration [15].

It has also been demonstrated that loneliness, social support, stressful situations such as exams, personality variables, etc., have been studied. The treatments carried out have shown certain effectiveness, these being mainly: Visualization techniques, Directed Imagination, Relaxation, Cognitive-Behavioral Stress Control Techniques, as well as Meditation, Shamanic Techniques, Prayers, etc. Any of these techniques can be useful if it is practised with the necessary rigor, whatever the psychological approach used. However, relaxation produces physiological states that, combined with the representation of images (imagination), can become so-called meditation techniques, positive visualization, directed imagination, etc. That is to say, positive emotion, in this case pleasant, would be the combination of the body state with a mental representation in the form of an image and thought [15].

Furthermore, Bower in 2003 [16], developed a handy tool that achieved more significant control of emotions and cognitive processes called guided imagination. To develop desired changes in behavior, guided imagery can be used to relieve muscle tension, reduce or eliminate pain, and facilitate the process of managing stressful situations through behavioral change. In this technique, it is important to describe the positive physiological and psychological effects of imagining scenes.

Understanding the communications between the brain and the immune system at their most intimate levels will also help health professionals believe in their patients when they tell them that their beliefs in the recovery process, hope, and laughter make you feel good.

8. Psychoneuroimmunology in children

There are very few studies on interventions based on psychoneuroimmunology (PNI) in pediatric patients. Studies reported that inappropriate clinical settings, knowledge of PNI could improve outcomes for pediatric surgical patients. Additionally, parents who receive these same services may also experience better psychological health, allowing them to be more available and prepared to support their children's recovery [17].

Castes in 1999 [18], carried out an investigation in the Isla de Coche, Venezuela, entitled: "Clinical, immunological changes associated with a psychosocial support program based on psychoneuroimmunology in asthmatic children", the authors state that anatomical evidence is presented, physiological and functional that demonstrate the interaction between the central nervous system (CNS), the endocrine system and the immune system. Likewise, it is shown that this communication is bidirectional, and the scientific bases that establish communication between the immune system and the CNS are provided. Likewise, the relationship between stress and the immune response is pointed out. We also present the results of our group that show that a psychosocial intervention based on psychoneuroimmunology (PNI) produced a significant decrease ($p < 0.05$) in the number of asthmatic attacks and the consumption of inhaled b2 agonist, together with a significant improvement ($p < 0.05$) of lung function (FEV1), when compared before the PNI intervention. A significant decrease was also found in specific IgE antibodies against Ascaris lumbricoides and in the marker CD23 (low-affinity receptor for IgE) post-intervention. In contrast, a significant increase ($p < 0.001$) of NK cells (CD56) and T cells with the receptor for IL-2 (CD25) was found after PNI intervention. None of these significant changes was found in children in the non-operated control group. These results demonstrate that the PNI intervention induces immunological alterations that are probably responsible for the clinical and physiological improvements observed in the group under study.

In summary, these studies were able to demonstrate that the disease process and the quality of life of a child can present favorable changes as a result of the application of a psychological intervention protocol based on psychoneuroimmunology, which systematically contains activities that allow the patient to work on the awareness of their disease and exercise active participation in their self-healing.

8.1 Psychoneuroimmunology intervention protocol for children with cancer

The authors developed a psychological intervention protocol based on psychoneuroimmunology principles for children with leukemia, and it was published in 2019 [19]; given its proven effectiveness at the research level, we allow ourselves to show its structure in detail.

It is a structured programme aimed at children between 5 and 15 years of age diagnosed with leukemia. A total of 30 pediatric patients with the diagnosis of acute lymphoblastic leukemia were evaluated. The BFM chemotherapy treatment protocol (Berlin-Frankfurt-Münster, 2009) was applied to the entire sample. From the sample, 18 patients were assigned to the experimental group. The psychoneuroimmunology-based psychological intervention protocol was applied during the remission induction period, and 12 children who belonged to the control group did not receive said protocol.

This protocol consists of different activities grouped together to psycho-educate the child and achieve learning about his illness, medical treatment and the influence of her emotions on his Immune System. The protocol has a printed and digital didactic story (audiobook) called “A Battle Won, My Fight Against Leukemia”. It is made up of four chapters: Knowing my body, now I know what is happening to me, my treatment and the power of my mind. Likewise, an activities notebook is included to verify the knowledge that the child has acquired, including the development of activities that motivate and reinforce the knowledge that the patient must have to face their disease and complete their oncology treatment successfully physically and mentally.

Play therapy in psychoneuroimmunology aims to give the child the opportunity to become familiar with stimuli or objects of interest in the disease process or interact with objects symbolically loaded with medical content to stimulate thoughts and fantasies about the procedures be performed, which will be submitted.

Among the playful techniques used is drawing, since it allows the individual to externally represent how he imagines his disease, the immune system and its treatment, among others. These actions allow the therapist to evaluate the perception that he is having in a conscious or unconscious way of the disease and treatment experience.

For this reason the Program is complemented with playful strategies, employing puppets representing the immune system, a memory game referring to the psychoeducational story "A Battle Won, My Fight Against Leukaemia." These strategies seek to maintain the child's attention and interest in learning and know more about her body and consolidate the story's informative content and the manual (see table by phases).

Objective	Session No.	Strategy / Activity	Procedure
Provide information to the patient around their body, specifically about the function of their bone marrow, through recreational activities adjusted to their evolutionary development.	Session 1	Personal History - 1st Part Activity Notebook	Encourage the writing of their own story about the onset of the disease.
		Cover of your personal story	Encourage the realization of the cover of your story.
		Draw your bone marrow	Encourage the child to draw his blood factory.
		Draw your platelets	Encourage the child to capture how he imagines his platelet battalion, stimulate the importance of using his imagination.
	Session 2	Alphabet soup	Indicate the search for words in the alphabet soup. Provide help and review the meaning of each word.
		Draw your red blood cells	Encourage the child to capture how he imagines his oxygen battalion, stimulate the importance of using his imagination.
		Draw your white blood cells	Encourage the child to capture how he imagines his white blood cells, highlight the importance of using his imagination.
Psychoeducation to the patient about his disease: Leukemia	Session 3	Questions of interest	Allow the use of their own expressions and ideas.
		Draw your Hospital	Encourage the patient to draw a picture of the hospital, allow him the space to express what he likes about the Institution.
		Name or draw the people who support you in your treatment.	Encourage the child to capture through drawing the people who accompany him during his treatment.
		Complete the next phrases	Guide the patient to respond correctly
		Draw the Blastos	Encourage the child to capture how he imagines the blasts, encourage the importance of using her imagination.
Psychoeducation to the patient in relation to the oncological treatment of Leukemia	Session 4	Some questions of interest	Tell the child or adolescent the questions to answer.

Objective	Session No.	Strategy / Activity	Procedure
		Draw how the QT works	Encourage the child to use her experience and capture how he imagines QT acting on his body
		Draw the professional team	Encourage the patient to draw the medical personnel accompanying him during treatment. Provide a space to express your thoughts
		Coloring your friends the medicines	Encourage creative use
		Draw yourself receiving QT	Encourage the child to use her experience and draw himself receiving his cancer treatment.
Psychoeducation to the child about his immune system and the influence of emotions in his battle against Leukemia.	Session 5	Some questions of interest	Tell the child or adolescent the questions to answer.
		put the words in order	Point out to the child that with the use of her imagination he can draw what her illness is like inside her body.
		Draw the disease	Encourage the child to use her imagination and draw what her active defense system is like in her body
	Session 6	Draw your immune system	Encourage the child to use her imagination and draw how she imagines her neutrophils. It is important to rely on playful material (dolls or puppets)
		Draw your neutrophils	Stimulate the patient imagine and draw their B Lymphocytes. It is important to rely on playful material (dolls or puppets)
		Draw your B Lymphocytes	Give directions for the completion of these activities and motivate him to express his knowledge about these characters: Mac, Lympho T, Lympho B.
		Link the dots	Stimulate the patient to imagine and draw the immunological battle in her body, allow her to narrate it and translate it into the Manual
		Complete the drawing	Allow the child space to express how he imagines himself totally healthy, relate the activities that he visualizes doing to draw in the manual.

At the end of the Psychoeducation, the phase of guided imagination based on psychoneuroimmunology continues, which is programmed in an important phase of the child's medical treatment protocol for day 33 for patients with Acute Lymphoid Leukemia according to the ALL Protocol. IC-BFM 2009.

For the guided imagination phase, the authors created audio, intending to relax and take an imaginary journey in your body to activate your immune system and thus activate your healing process. These exercises were carried out in the hospital and at home. A record was made daily and was complemented with didactic activities where the child could capture visualizations of her within her body through drawing.

This phase is accompanied by an information session for parents that reinforces the importance of psychoneuroimmunology techniques and the importance of them being involved in the treatment of the child and motivating them to carry out relaxation sessions at home.

Variables	Dimensios	Subdimensions	Indicators	Measurement
ILLNESS PROCESS	Immunological parameters	Lymphocyte population	Total Lymphocytes Natural killer T lymphocyte B lymphocyte	Peripheral blood analysis by flow cytometry.
		Lymphocyte subpopulation	CD4, CD8	Peripheral blood analysis by flow cytometry.
		Immunoglobulins	IgA, IgM, IgG	Peripheral blood analysis in clinical laboratory.
	Clinical parameters	Hospitalization	Days of Hospitalized stay Frequency of hospital admissions. Induction duration	Clinical History Record
		Signs and symptom	Fever Pain Skin paleness Vomiting Liquid Evacuations Hyporexia Dyspnoea Tachycardia Lymphadenopathy Signs of Bleeding Hepatosplenomegaly	Clinical History Record
		Complications during the induction phase	Febrile neutropenia Mucositis Diabetes Septic shock Bronchial hyperactivity Pneumonia Phlebitis Enterocolitis Convulsive syndrome Others	Clinical History Record
	Pharmacological parameters	Medication and support administration	Medicines Antibiotics Analgesic Pain Therapy Antipyretic Antiemetic	Clinical History Record

Variables	Dimensios	Subdimensions	Indicators	Measurement
			Supportive Therapy: Colony Stimulating Factor Globular (Blood) Transfusion Platelet transfusion Parental nutrition Respiratory therapies	

To evaluate the disease process, the immunological, clinical, and pharmacological parameters in the child are considered during the induction phase of chemotherapy treatment by recording medical records during hospitalization and laboratory tests for Immunoglobulins Lymphocytes and subpopulation of Lymphocytes by cytometry (See below table).

To evaluate the Quality of Life: It is obtained by applying the Quality Questionnaire in Pediatric Oncology by Jordi Bernabeu, standardized in the applied child population (2014). The dimensions of the Questionnaire were

- Social functioning.
- Symptoms.
- Autonomy
- School performance.
- Psychological discomfort.
- Psychological well-being.

8.2 Results to highlight from the research

The results of the study indicate that the intervention protocol based on psychoneuroimmunology (PNI) positively modified the clinical evolution (symptoms and treatment) of the patients, substantially improved their immune parameters and significantly increased the quality of life of children with cancer, specifically in a sample of children with acute lymphoblastic leukemia.

Summary of the effects of the Psychological Intervention based on PNI

Clinical Parameters		
Signs and symptoms	Fever	↓ ↓
	Pain	O
	Skin paleness	O
	Vomiting	O
	Liquid stools	O
	Hyperoxia	O
	Dyspnoea	O

Clinical Parameters		
	Tachycardia	O
	Lymphadenopathy	O
	Signs of Bleeding	O
	Hepatosplenomegaly	O
Complications	Febrile neutropenia	O
	Pneumonia Phlebitis Enterocolitis Convulsive syndrome Others	O
	Mucositis	O
	Phlebitis	O
	Diabetes	O
	Enterocolitis	O
	Septic shock	O
	Convulsive syndrome	O
	Bronchial hyperactivity	O
	Others	O
Pharmacological and support parameters		
Medicines	Pain Therapy Antibiotics Antipyretic Antiemetic	↓
	Antibiotics Antipyretic Antiemetic	↓
	Antipyretic	↓
	Antiemetic	O
Support therapy	Colony Stimulating Factor	O
	Globular (Blood) Transfusion	O
	Platelet transfusion	O
	Parenteral nutrition	O
	Respiratory Therapies	↓
Immune parameters		
Lymphocyte population	Natural Killer	↑
	T lymphocyte	↑
	B lymphocyte	↑
Lymphocyte subpopulation	CD4	↑
	CD8	↑
Immunoglobulins	IgM IgA	↑
	IgA	↑
	IgG	O
Quality of life		↑

↑ ↓	Statistically significant difference
O	No statistically significant differences

8.3 Some effects of the intervention protocol based on psychoneuroimmunology on clinical parameters

8.3.1 Symptoms and signs

In this regard, the PNI-based intervention protocol's efficacy was directly appreciated in its clinical picture, especially the symptoms and signs compatible with infectious and inflammatory processes secondary to chemotherapy; Among these, statistically significant differences stand out on the days with fever during the induction process. The operated group had six days less fever than the control group. There was a lower frequency of vomiting, dyspnea and tachycardia in the operated patients than the controls; Although these differences did not reach statistical significance due to the values' variance, they could be taken as likely trends in a larger sample of patients.

8.3.2 Complications during the induction phase

The intervened group had a tendency (statistically not significant) to a lower frequency of complications during the induction phase, especially those of an infectious type such as febrile neutropenia, mucositis, septic shock, pneumonia, abscesses, chickenpox and enterocolitis. However, although there was no apparent effect on the duration of some symptoms of an infectious nature, the need to use antibiotics for fewer days in those treated - as described below - suggests that these processes were less severe or easier to manage.

8.4 Effects of the intervention protocol based on psychoneuroimmunology on pharmacological parameters

According to the results, although there was an improvement in the clinical evolution, it was not reflected in fewer days of hospitalization, if it was consistently associated with a lower frequency in the use of treatments to control fever and infectious and inflammatory processes: antibiotics, antipyretics, pain therapy and respiratory therapies in the intervened group compared to controls.

There was evidence to support the view that the lower use of antibiotics in operated patients was related to improved cellular immunity, although not humoral. The use of antibiotics was linearly and inversely correlated with a higher number of CD8 T lymphocytes and NK cells, mediators of cellular immunity, but not with the number of B lymphocytes, which participate in humoral immunity.

On the other hand, in the study, three variables estimated pain: directly, days with pain as a symptom (clinical parameter) and indirectly, days of pain therapy and days with analgesics (treatment parameters). A tendency to report pain for a smaller number of days was observed in those operated on than controls, although this difference did not reach statistical significance. However, the number of days during which pain therapy was administered was significantly lower in patients concerning controls. This suggests that the psychotherapeutic intervention markedly influenced the sensory function of leukemia patients during chemotherapy induction.

8.4.1 Supportive therapy

It was observed that the operated patients required respiratory therapy for 82% shorter periods than the controls. This smaller statistically significant difference in the intervened group may be due to a greater recurrence of infections that required this type of support for their recovery.

It was also evidenced that the intervened patients required colony growth factor therapies for periods 50% shorter than the controls. However, statistical significance was not reached due to the wide variability of the control group. However, this finding suggests that the intervened group presented a lower level of leukopenia during this period, as it required less use of this pharmacological agent.

8.5 Effects of the intervention protocol based on psychoneuroimmunology on immune parameters

Significant changes in the immune parameters' values, both cellular and humoral, were observed during the induction process in pediatric patients with acute lymphoblastic leukemia. These changes suggest that the better clinical evolution of the operated patients was linked to a substantial improvement in their immune function.

8.5.1 Cellular immunity

Specifically, there was a significant increase in the number of natural killers NK cells and CD8 and CD4 type T lymphocytes in the intervened group, especially at the end of the chemotherapy induction period (day 64), compared to the control group.

It is important to remember that both natural killer cells or NK cells and T lymphocytes are involved in cellular immunity mechanisms against neoplastic cells. Within the T lymphocytes population, there are two subpopulations of lymphocytes, CD4 and CD8, both of great clinical importance. CD4 lymphocytes act mainly against parasites, bacteria and fungi, and to a lesser degree, against viruses and tumor antigens, while CD8 lymphocytes will act mainly against tumor cells and viruses. Therefore, a more significant number of natural killer NK cells and CD8 lymphocytes, specialized in the destruction of malignant cells, in children treated with the protocol based on psychoneuroimmunology implied an improvement in their cellular immunity, and as a result, a lower frequency of infectious symptoms, which led to less need for antibiotics and antipyretics in the children treated in this study.

8.5.2 Humoral immunity

Serum levels of IgM and IgA antibodies were significantly higher in the intervened group in relation to the control group, which suggests that the PNI-based intervention increased humoral immunity. It is important to remember that B lymphocytes are immunocompetent cells whose primary function is to produce antibodies, a specific type of protein called immunoglobulins. Thus, it can be assumed that the higher serum antibody levels in the operated children were significantly related to the increase in the number of B lymphocytes.

8.6 Effect of the intervention protocol based on psychoneuroimmunology on quality of life

The recovery of quality of life was significantly greater in the operated patients than in the controls. This was linked to an improvement in both clinical symptoms and immunological parameters. It is important to highlight that this recovery of quality of life was linearly and positively correlated with the number of NK cells and CD8 lymphocytes, suggesting that an immunological substrate made this change possible.

9. Psychoneuroimmunology: present and future in clinical and health practice

The amount of research that reports the mind–body expresses that there is no longer any doubt about this relationship since its biochemical mechanism is recognized. That is why health professionals' objective is to encourage the promotion of developing health plans that incorporate psychoneuroimmunology techniques and promote the reduction of psychosocial risk factors.

On the other hand, it is exposed that Psychoneuroimmunology gives us the understanding of the mental factors that modulate the immune system, offering a transdisciplinary perspective of the way of understanding health and disease. This leads us to reflect on the need to incorporate public health measures considering these aspects and the challenges and opportunities for researchers and teachers in the health area to promote training and treatment programs oriented to these findings.

The consideration of Psychoneuroimmunology in understanding the disease is also of high impact in the prevention and proposals of public health policies, considering the high levels of stress to which children and adults are subjected in some harmful environments.

The information presented here wants to be a great incentive to promote mechanisms that integrate all disciplines within the academic, governmental, clinical and health sectors to generate policies and mutual support to develop plans that promote health and influence the healing of diseases on a physical and mental level.

10. Conclusion

Psychoneuroimmunology has provided a clear scientific insight into the mind–body relationship. This knowledge allows an integrative view of both prevention and treatment of diseases, representing a significant challenge. Research has shown the evident influence of stress and other psychological factors that can affect health through interactions with the immune, endocrine and nervous systems. This has provided a solid evidence base and has also improved our understanding of people's central role in their healing, both for adults and children, which implies both recovery of their physical condition and their quality of life.

Acknowledgements

Special thanks to Dr. Marianela Cástes, pioneer of psychoneuroimmunology in Latin America, researcher and main personal inspiration at the PNI level.

To Dr. Rosario Montilva, pediatric oncologist and Coordinator of the Pediatric Oncology Unit of the Pediatric Specialties Hospital, and to the entire team: Dr. Betty Urdaneta de Ramos (Hematologist), Dr. Fatima Viloria (Pediatric Oncologist), Dr. Yoleida Colmenares (Pediatric Oncologist), Lic. Leila Nouheid (Nutritionist), Lic Maira Alvarez and Mayra Vargas, both committed nurses.

Special thanks to the children and family members of the Pediatric Specialties Hospital, who participated in the research and who continue to be active in putting forth the greatest force to heal.

Author details

Margarita del Valle Chacin Fuenmayor[1*] and Josymar Chacin de Fernandez[2]

1 Horley Psychology and Shineeq, Horley, United Kingdom

2 Avantem, San José, Costa Rica

*Address all correspondence to: margarita@horleypsychology.co.uk

References

[1] Engel, G. L. The need for a new medical model: A challenge for biomedicine. Science. 1977; 196, 129–136.

[2] Solomon, G.F., Segerstrom, S.G., Grohr, P., Kemeny, M., and Fahey, J. Shaking up immunity: psychological and immunologic changes following a natural disaster. Psychosomatic Medicine 1997; 59, 114-127.

[3] Fleshner, M. , Laudenslager, M. L. , Simons, L. , & Maier, S. F. Reduced serum antibodies associated with social defeat in rats. Physiology & Behavior, 1989, 45, 1183-1187.

[4] Alford, L., Findings of interest from immunology and psychoneuroimmunology. Manual therapy, 2007, 10.1016/j. math.2006.06.007

[5] Vidal, J. Psiconeuroinmunología. Barcelona: Ediciones de la Universidad de Barcelona. 2006

[6] Ortega, MC. La Psiconeuroinmunología y La Promoción de la Salud. Universidad Nacional de Educación a Distancia, 2011.

[7] Lyubomirsky, S., et al. The benefits of frequent positive affect: Does happiness lead to success? Psychological Bulletin, 131, (6), 2005, 803-855.

[8] Maruso, S. M. . El laboratorio del alma. Historias para sanar que merecen ser contadas. Buenos Aires: Ediciones B; 2009.

[9] Oblitas, L. Encyclopedia of Health Psychology. Bogotá: PSICOM. 2007

[10] Bradlyn, A. S.; Pollock, B. H. Quality of life research in the Pediatric Oncology Group. Journal of the National Cancer Institute. 1996; 20: 49-53

[11] Parsons, S K; Barlow, S E; Levy, S L; Supran, S E; Kaplan, S H (1999). Health-relates quality of life in pediatric bone marrow transplant survivors: according to whom?. International journal of cancer 12: 46-51

[12] Antoni, MH. Stress Management Effects on Psychological, Endocrinological, and Immune Functioning in Men with HIV Infection: Empirical Support for a Psychoneuroimmunological Model. Stress: The International Journal on the Biology of Stress, 2003; 6, 173-188.

[13] Robinson, FP. (2002). Psycho-endocrine-immune response to mindfulness-based stress reduction in HIV-infected individuals. Dissertation Abstracts International: Section- B: The Sciences and Engineering, 63(1-B), 179.

[14] Lutgendorf, S & Costanzo, E (2003) Psychoneuroinmunology and health psychology. An integrative model. Brain, Behavior and Inmunity. 17, 225-232.

[15] Ramos, V., Rivero Burón, R., Piqueras J. A., García, L. J. & Oblitas, L. A. Psiconeuroinmunología: Conexiones Entre Sistema Nervioso Y Sistema Inmune. Suma Psicológica, 2008; 15(1) 115-141.

[16] Bower JE, Kemeny ME, Taylor SE, et al. Finding positive meaning and its association with natural killer cell cytotoxicity among participants in a bereavement-related disclosure intervention. Annals of Behavioral Medicine. 2003; 25: 146–155.

[17] Tagge, E. P., Natali, E. L., Lima, E., Leek, D., Neece, C. L., & Randall, K. F. Psychoneuroimmunology and the pediatric surgeon. Seminars in Pediatric Surgery. 2013; 22(3), 144–148.

[18] Castes, M; Hagel, I., Palenque, M., Canelones, P., Corao, A and Lynch, N. Immunological changes associated with

clinica improvement of asthmatic children submitted to psycho-social intervention. Brain, Behavior and Immunity. 1999; 13, 1 -13

[19] Chacin-Fernández J, Chacin Fuenmayor M, Piñerua-Shuhaibar L, Suarez-Roca H. Psychological intervention based on psychoneuroimmunology improves clinical evolution, quality of life, and immunity of children with leukemia: A preliminary study. Health Psychol Open. 2019 Apr 1;6(1): 2055102919838902. doi: 10.1177/ 2055102919838902.

Section 3

Quality of Life in the Context of the Social Gradient and Social Determinants of Health

Chapter 7

Poverty and Social Psychology: The Importance of Integrative Manner

Filiz Çömez Polat

Abstract

As one of the most important social problems in the world, poverty has been studied by various disciplines. Although poverty is a basic subject of economics, it has also become one of the prominent research fields of social sciences in recent years. Poverty also relates to many psychological processes and mechanisms just as in the other social problems in the world. It is assumed that the social-psychological approach to poverty may contribute to establishing different road maps in combating poverty. Therefore this study aims at contributing to poverty reduction efforts from the social-psychological point of view by providing an integrative review of the social psychological correlates of poverty based on the empirical findings. Also, by including arguments such as social identity, migration, ideology and social context in poverty studies to be conducted with a social psychological perspective, a contribution can be made to poverty reduction with multidimensional research methods.

Keywords: poverty, psychological processes, poverty reduction, integrative manner, qualitative research, quantitative research

1. Introduction

Poverty has been increasing in parallel with globalization, which is characterized by rapid technological developments and different political and economic balances [1]. Although there are aspects of information and technology that facilitate human life, these advances do not bring the same prosperity for everyone. It is known that not everyone lives equally well or easily, and some masses lack even the basic needs. Therefore, poverty is a phenomenon that affects large social groups, and its individual and social consequences have been tried to be overcome.

There are numerous studies on poverty and combating poverty. These studies generally focused on the definition of poverty, economic analysis, and economic effects of poverty with globalization and social rights [2–9]. According to the general definition, poverty refers to the deprivation of economic, material, and cultural resources, and the deprivation of welfare [10, 11]. While another definition of poverty describes poverty as a permanent or temporary lack of quality, technical, physical strength, intellectual ability, freedom, and individual dignity [12], different types of poverty are also mentioned in the literature, such as female poverty, child poverty, urban–rural poverty, etc. [13]. Consequently, poverty has multiple dimensions, and diverse effects, and it might be addressed regarding its economic, political, individual, and social basis [14–17].

IntechOpen

For psychological inquiry, it seems crucial to make a distinction between the two different conceptualizations of poverty in order understand psychological aspects of poverty: absolute poverty and relative poverty [18–20]. Absolute poverty is defined as the state in which individuals do not afford to buy their basic needs, and the inability of the household or individual to attain the minimum welfare level that can sustain their lives. In other words, absolute poverty refers to the deprivation of basic human needs, which usually includes food, water, hygiene, clothing, shelter, healthcare, and education [21]. This definition indicates the inadequacy of material/economic resources and accepts everyone who is below certain standards as poor wherever they are in the world [22]. The data showed that over 1 billion of the approximately 2.8 billion poor in the world live in absolute poverty (living with an income of less than $ 1–1.5 per day according to World Bank) [23]. On the other hand, relative poverty refers to the state in which individuals are below a certain rate of the average welfare level of the society and have been spending below a certain limit according to the general level of the society [24]. Relative poverty is related to the unequal distribution of resources or power in a society in which some people lack the adequate resources to live in the standard they desire, while others do not [18]. Therefore, relative poverty is based on economic inequality in society, which exists largely and persistently all around the world. In addition to the material disadvantages and economic insecurity, relative poverty has some severe social-psychological consequences, such as reduced self-esteem, feelings of disrespect, and humiliation [25–27].

From the different definitions and forms of poverty mentioned above, one can ask that who are these individuals who are absolutely and relatively poor? A poor person is usually described as the one who cannot have sufficient economic resources to buy basic needs [28–30]. Poor people are also defined referring to Lewis's [31] concept of "culture of poverty". The "culture of poverty", which is learned in the family and tends to be passed down from generation to generation, includes normative patterns acquired by the poor as a group rather than from the economic side [10, 31]. In other words, poverty culture points to a common set of attitudes and behaviors that develop depending on the conditions [32]. But we cannot say that "every poor has the characteristics of poverty culture". It may change depending on the culture, historical, and economic context and from person to person. In other words, the person might be "poor" according to the official criteria, but may not perceive himself/herself as poor when he/she compares himself/herself to "another individuals or groups who are poorer. And also, a poor society may not have the characteristics of a culture of poverty mentioned above (see also [33, 34]). This situation shows that social sciences should discuss poverty as a multidimensional construct with its different aspects/results and processes. Although individual perceptions are not sufficient in understanding the dynamics of poverty, the interaction between individual perceptions and societal values and norms should be taken into account. Therefore, this review paper aims to present social psychological findings within a theoretical framework in an integrative manner. The distinctive feature of this study is that it considers poverty as a "process", rather than a psychological "situation". The association of the information resulting from the handling of the psychological processes in a multidimensional or integrative methodological manner with the steps to be taken towards poverty alleviation indicates the methodical framework of this study. The proposed framework also emphasizes the continuity of the interrelation of psychological and socio-political processes. It is shown below in **Figure 1**.

This study aims to rethink the shortcomings of approaches analyzing poverty, poverty processes, and integrative methodological framework. In other words, this study underlines that social psychology should approach poverty analyzes in an integrative manner. So, it strives to emphasize a social psychological understanding

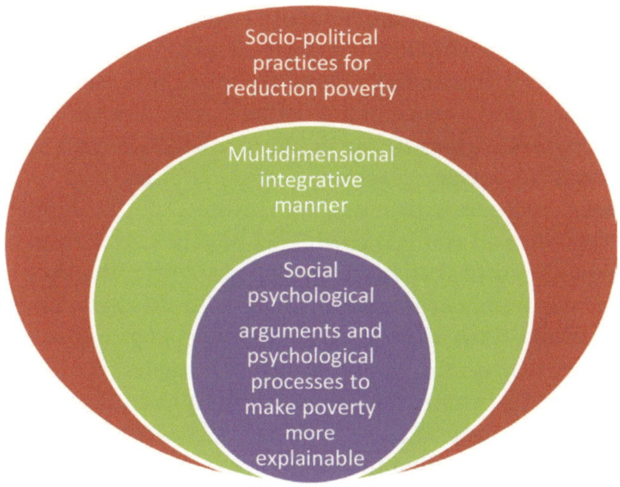

Figure 1.
The analytical framework for the social psychological assessment of poverty.

that can establish relations with different disciplines to eliminate the poverty problem. In this context, it is a literature review study that focuses on the shortcomings of the methodological and theoretical stance of social psychology in poverty studies, rather than a direct critical approach. It is also explained why existing social psychological approaches to the aforementioned deficiencies and poverty do not contribute to overcoming the poverty problem. The integrative approach proposed as an alternative to these explanations; and how and in what direction the steps to be taken towards poverty alleviation can be guided.

Two questions related to the purpose and methodological stance of this review has been determined: (1) which social psychological arguments make poverty more explainable? And (2) what role does the proposed integrative approach to poverty analysis play in ending poverty and how is this new analytical framework set up? To find answers to these questions, firstly, previous studies about poverty in social psychology literature will be explained. Afterward, a discussion will be held on how to establish an integrative approach that can guide poverty to make it clearer and eliminate it.

2. Previous social psychological accounts of poverty

When we look at the relationship between psychology and poverty, we see three major study routes. These routes are causal attributions of poverty, personality characteristics of the poor, and psychological outcomes of poverty [35]. Several studies were conducted on social psychological perspective are often intended to establish individual characteristics or attributions by others of how poor people look or who they are [36, 37].

2.1 Causal attributions of poverty

The area on which social psychology focuses mostly is poverty attributions [3, 36–46]. The ways of explaining poverty and the perceived causes of poverty are frequently studied regarding causal attributions on poverty in social psychology [47]. Causal attributions of poverty are generally evaluated in three dimensions: individual, structural and fatalistic. Individual attributions include lack of effort, failure, and laziness of the poor; structural attributions focus on the social and economical system and the state policies; and lastly, fatalistic attributions refer to bad luck and fate [48]. Feagin [49] found that in the United States people had attributed poverty to individual factors to a great extent (53%), and structural factors (22%). Fatalistic factors were the least attributed factor (18%) when explaining the causes of poverty. It was also claimed that the structural factors are two-dimensional rather than being a single dimension: "economic-structural" (low wages, lack of job opportunities) and "bias-structural" (prejudice and discrimination against the poor, lower wages for women) [50].

In another study Birdsall and Hamovdi [38] in which structural causes are synthesized together with cultural attributes, the economic and administrative foundations that cause poverty were evaluated through cultural characteristics. When we look at the causal attributions of poverty in different geographies/cultures, we come across different results. Hine and Mouitel [48] investigated the attributed causes of poverty comparing Canadian and Filipino participants. They found that the Canadian participants attributed poverty to natural causes (climate, location) and the conflict, while Filipinos tended to blame the poor and poverty itself. Besides, different groups within the same cultural setting were found to tend to explain the causes of poverty (i.e. liberals emphasized structural and social factors more frequently than conservatives). Similarly, Solak and Göregenli [47] showed that the poverty attributions have three dimensions in Turkey: individual (personal responsibility, hardworking and personal effort), structural and fatalistic. Moreover, migration emerged as another factor that was attributed as a cause of poverty in this study. In other words, the "rural to urban migration process" is pointed to as the cause of poverty. It is discussed in section 3.2 below that migration is a factor that needs to be discussed in detail, rather than a causal attribution in social psychology studies. Although these studies investigate poverty from different ideological and structural perspectives, the focus of all is the same: the causes of poverty. Exploring the causal attributions for poverty may contribute to poverty reduction but it would fall short of explaining the social psychological processes and the dynamic interaction between individual and social-structural factors that underlie poverty [34].

2.2 Poverty as a process

In the literature, there are criticisms towards approaches that point out that poverty is a situation rather than a dynamic process and there are opinions that psychology remains "indifferent" in combating poverty (see also [51]). Accordingly, although poverty constitutes an important subject on which psychologists have focused directly for a considerable amount of time, the majority of studies have taken the form of an individual-level analysis, and have usually failed to take into account interactional, contextual, and hierarchical aspects. For instance, focusing on the poor as separate individuals, such as emphasizing their attributes as being passive, leads eventually to appointing blame to the poor themselves for the situation from which they suffer [34]. There are also opinions that poverty takes up a little place in social psychology, assuming that it is a subject that does not attract much attention and has no "popularity" (see also [52, 53]). Lemieux and Pratto [54] argue that social relations in the allocation of economic resources, and therefore the phenomenon such as violence, prejudices, social dominance, and discrimination play a role in the continuation of poverty. For this reason, we should focus on social psychological processes in the understanding of poverty and contextual relationships that cause poverty to continue. In this regard, psychological dynamics and processes associated with poverty seem crucial as they would provide clues about the solution of the problem and contribute to the theoretical explanation of poverty from a social psychological perspective. Also, the studies of the psychological process can provide foresight to what complementary arguments are needed in social psychology's discourse and its suggestions for combating poverty.

Psychological processes may be related to the way the poor perceive themselves. A study with blue-collar participants working in different sectors (e.g. working as taxi drivers, doormen, cleaners) in Turkey was asked to define "who the poor is" [8]. Results indicated that they define poor as those who live in worse conditions than themselves. Consistent with their poor definition they did not perceive themselves as poor when they compared themselves with the poorer. Besides, the study showed that one out of every three people in Turkey (77%) believed that poverty is overcome by individual efforts. Another study directly addressed poor people and investigated their subjective perceptions on poverty in the framework of Social Identity Theory (Tajfel and Turner, [55] (Akfırat et al. [34]. In this study, it was found that the strategies to cope with poverty by poor people change as a function of whether they acknowledge that they were a part of the poor group, and whether they perceive poverty as changeable and illegitimate. Specifically, the results show that poor people who did not perceive themselves as poor, though they were poor according to official criteria, preferred creative and individual strategies to get rid of poverty.

In a similar vein, Jetten and Peter [56] discuss the role of social identity, social comparison, power, and ideological relations and group dynamics that help to understand economic inequality. The authors concluded that it is necessary to emphasize specific group dynamics for different societies in terms of economic inequality and poverty. There are also studies explaining that an unequal socio-economic structure increases social comparison between individuals and groups, reveals competition, and some groups seek self-esteem [57–59]. It is seen that these studies which predict that economic inequality can have harmful psychological consequences focus on the importance of social comparison processes. The system that allows people to think that they will have beter living conditions if they spend more effort individually make people compare themselves with those who are in better conditions. However, in most cases, poverty is independent of individual effort. Therefore when people do not reach the desired conditions they tend to blame themselves.

Xiemenes et al. [60] focus on the perception of poverty in the frame of community psychology, the historical and social background of poverty in the context of Brazil and Latin American countries were investigated. The researchers pointed out the roles of migration, slavery, and violence in the emergence and perpetuation of poverty. Thus, the importance of historical-cultural background in understanding and combating poverty were emphasized. The researchers also mentioned the need for examining poverty on academic-social and political grounds, and the importance of knowing the poor population well, determining their needs and, taking political steps to provide better conditions. Guzzo [61] also emphasizes that psychological inquiry should focus on the political attitude when combating poverty. On the other hand, Okoroji et al. [62] prioritize the importance of the social-psychological analysis of marginalization towards the poor addressing the relationship of poverty with the representations produced in the media and politics is expressed. Many studies that focus on the multidimensional evaluation of poverty also point to suggestions for reducing or ending poverty. Especially in index studies created through data collected from different countries contain the effects of emergent conditions such as COVID-19 [63, 64]. From this point of view, it emerges that these emergent conditions and psychological processes should be evaluated from a socio-political perspective.

2.3 Outcomes of poverty

We have said that the psychological approach to poverty generally focuses on the possible consequences of poverty and marks poverty as a "condition" [51]. The first psychological study on the consequences of poverty was Lewis' [65] work in which he explained the particular behavioral patterns of the poor that are transmitted down from generation to generation through socialization processes. It means that the values and behaviors of the poor become determinants of the lower socio-economic status. Some studies have focused on the personality characteristics and traits of the poor such as lack of entrepreneurial personality, lack of participation in political and association activities, lack of purpose towards career goal [35, 66–68]. Some other works investigated the effects of poverty on emotions, cognitive skills, and mental health [69–77].

Research shows that other than the material difficulties, being poor is also associated with stigma, feelings of worthlessness, and it is negatively related to individual well-being [59, 72, 78–81]. For example, Moussa-Smona [80] found that economically vulnerable people have a lower level of subjective well-being and life satisfaction than those who are more secure. Similarly, Okoroji et al. [62] showed that stigmatization processes produced by representations in media and politics make poor people suffer from marginalization, which in turn causes vulnerability for psychological distress. Another study demonstrates that social injustice and poverty increases negative child experiences [82]. Some other studies focus on poverty in third- world countries which point to similar negative psychological outcomes (see also [83, 84]).

While there has been robust evidence that poverty reduces the indicators of well-being, some scholars discuss that focusing on negative individual outcomes might buffer the efforts of reducing poverty. Such a state is conceptualized as a "poverty trap" in which an individual believes that s/he cannot escape unless an extremely large change takes place, such as a dramatic improvement in their economic situation (see also [85]) [51, 86, 87]. According to another critical approach, negative outcome oriented-research reinforces the prejudices and stereotypes imposed on the poor and points to anger or accusatory feelings. The psychology of being poor and the mental and behavioral patterns that may arise in both adults and children as a result of poverty are the basis of these studies.

3. Discussion and conclusion

Traditional psychological works related to poverty have been criticized as being reductionist and individualistic, and as being far from discussing its contextual dimensions [88, 89]. Connolly [90] states that psychological studies that analyze the perception of poverty should be analyzed not only to environmental factors but also to include genetic, physical, familial, social, political factors. Carr and Sloan [91] argue that social psychological studies on poverty can be developed to be part of a global effort to reduce poverty without pathologizing poverty. In another word, psychological studies that can show the ability to progress in line with a global awareness in combating poverty should be increased. Yet, studies that focus solely on poor people can buffer the efforts to combat poverty and may prevent the multi-dimensional analysis of poverty. Therefore, social-psychological findings that can help develop strategies seem important rather than initiatives that can limit our understanding of both poverty and the poor [92]. At this point, it would be good to discuss the answer to the first question of this study (which social psychological arguments does poverty become more explainable?) that will provide a methodological framework. Below are the social-psychological arguments that should be included in the analysis and the suggestions:

3.1 Social psychological arguments and class-based approach

When the fact that poverty is ultimately a class-based problem juxtaposes with some of the arguments of social psychology, a significant contribution can be made to the literature. For example, social identity perception seems to be an argument that can make this contribution. **Social identity** and its arguments have a rich literature on the issue of poverty. It is possible to think about poverty with many arguments of Social Identity Theory [55] (such as social comparison, social mobility, intergroup conflict, in-group–/out-group perception). In this sense, poverty is a social category; It would not be wrong to point out poor individuals as a disadvantaged social identity. Departing from the process of different groups perceiving each other; class clues can be caught on the distinction between rich and poor. In other words; with the right questions to be asked for social comparison processes, class-level evaluation can be made. For example; with whom do the poor compare themselves and how do they perceive them? This question is important in two ways. It is important both in understanding the place of poor groups in the social hierarchy and in understanding how they evaluate the situation (poverty). In other words, it may be useful to discuss the perceptions of the poor as a group rather than the individuals. The economic conditions in which the individual lives, his/her contact with people living in better or worse conditions than himself, the existence of comparison groups (rich people) seem crucial in assessing his poverty situation [34]. That is, poor people's perception about their poverty may not be straightforward in the sense that she might categorize herself in the class system as the rich, the very rich, the poor, and the very poor depending on what groups she compares herself to. So, their perception of poverty does not change/changes or whether they see it legitimate or not can be revealed. It may be inevitable that the perception in question makes the distinction between the rich and the poor, which indicates income inequality, visible. In other words, it may be easier to handle the perception of being in a disadvantaged position within a class framework. And also, if we think together with the background of social identity theory; The question of which strategies (strategies to cope with disadvantage situation: individual, creative and collective) to choose to deal with poverty is also important. The question of why these strategies are preferred and which factors are effective in these preferences will also contribute to the research process. Therefore, rather than taking poverty as a static and stable phenomenon; the dynamic, political, class-based, and interactive account of poverty would provide a new basis for discussion on the poverty combating strategies. To add with the social identity perspective; the danger of **stigmatization** of the poor as an outgroup is also another responsibility for social psychologists. According to Fell and Hewstone [71], intergroup contact can be established to reduce stereotypes and prejudices in the context of in-group-outgroup perceptions, and thus self-efficacy perception of poor can develop. The purpose of providing communication/contact between groups requires focusing on social and psychological processes. As mentioned before, individual attributions-based studies on poverty may reinforce prejudices and stereotypes towards poor people. Starting from the idea that poverty is built or sustained through a social structure and social relations Perez et al. [93], a researcher should be aware of the scientific methodology used in his/her poverty research that may increase the negative effects of poverty.

Another area in which the class-based approach should be visible in poverty studies conducted with a social psychological perspective is related to **causal attributions.** We mentioned before the studies conducted on the causal attributions of poverty and the missing points of these studies. Learning the references to the causes of poverty will undoubtedly contribute to the field, but may not lead to steps to be taken to alleviate poverty. Therefore, as we mentioned above, it is to include the citations of the rich and the poor to the issue and try to understand why they need these citations. Because understanding the need in question will help us to reveal the discourses that perpetuate or legitimize poverty. The point that should be emphasized in the poverty attribution of people who are economically located in different classes is their perception of their position and how this perception reflects on their lives and language in practice. This point must be addressed together with a critical discursive stance on how the poverty discourse is constructed. And also, it will provide a broad perspective on how and why perceptions and causal attributions of poverty occur.

3.2 Arguments of social constructionist approach: social context, power relations, ideology

Harper [89] argued that a social constructionist approach would be more inclusive, focusing on the question of "how" in poverty studies. The social constructionist approach involves discourse analysis [94], discursive psychology [95, 96], critical discourse analysis [97, 98], and critical psychology [99]. And it is a multidisciplinary approach. Social constructionism emphasizes the common construction of knowledge in the world of understanding/interpretation that changes, transforms, and interprets according to the context and uses qualitative research methods methodologically [100]. In other words, people, events, and situations are all products of social processes. In this sense, it would be appropriate to focus on how it is formed in the mind and how it continues, rather than the subjective effect created by the perception of poverty. The question of how poverty is built in the minds of the rich and the poor take away from discussing poverty solely on an individual basis; referring to the representation of group members to the class level [98]. In other words, the problem of poverty is not only the subjective perceptions of individuals and their state of being affected by the situation; it also includes the power relations of being rich and poor. The emergence of power relations between groups; will remove the individual aspects of poverty associated with being strong and weak. In this way, the accusing, victimization, or discourses that perpetuate or legitimize the state of poverty attributed to the poor may decrease. Also, the legitimacy of the invisibility of the poor and therefore poverty in society, which are constantly positioned as victims, can be questioned. The questioning is revealed through the methodological process. Social constructionist methodology analyzes power-discourse and positioning in speech, focusing on the action of language [95]. Therefore, first of all, this perspective is needed to prevent the reproduction of the accusing language of the disadvantaged groups and to overturn the belief that "poverty is an ongoing-unchangeable phenomenon". The social constructionist approach reveals the language that sees poverty as "unchangeable" or "pathologizing"; can re-evaluate this language in terms of power and ideology relations. Discourse reproduces within ideology and establishes power relations through certain arguments (such as media, education, cultural-normative codes). For example, the social, cultural, ideological context in which poor people evaluate themselves and live, their interpretations of the state of poverty, how they position rich people, the basis or legitimate grounds of their strategies to cope with poverty, and how this process is in the context of ideological or power relations. In other words, knowing the cultural background of the geography in which we were born, the codes/norms of poverty, the daily language used for poor people or poverty, and providing suggestions in this context will make the research more powerful. And also, the question of how it is handled in society or through the media is important. Regarding the importance of this problem; We can give an example that how the poor/poverty is handled in the media affect both society's attitude towards poverty and policy- making [101]. Therefore, steps to be taken on a discursive basis to answer this question may also contribute to poverty reduction initiatives.

3.3 Gender

Why should social psychology include gender-related arguments as a variable in its analysis? The answer to this question aims to contribute to the production of egalitarian policies for the sexes (especially women) who experience poverty at different levels. Continuing learning since childhood can position women and men in different places in society; these positions frequently direct women to domestic work and men to jobs aimed at generating economic income. While examining the effects of poverty on the individual; The causes of poverty and gender-based inequalities become visible; gender-centered meaning worlds of poverty emerge [102]. The fact that female deprivation is becoming more pronounced compared to men seems to be related to the impact of socio-political processes and gender perspective (see also [103]). The relation in question regarding poverty and gender; Fertility, differences in wages, power relations within the household, and ongoing poverty between generations [104]. Explaining that women experience more poverty than men, female poverty, or feminization of deprivation is an argument that should be included in social psychological analysis. Studies focusing particularly on the gender impact on poverty; can also involve suggestions that lead to gender equality. These proposals are likely to contribute to political steps, especially to reduce women's poverty.

3.4 Migration

It is known that the phenomenon of migration in the literature has been shown by empirical studies as a feature attributed to the causes of poverty. But the approach that sees migration as a phenomenon causing poverty will be insufficient. We know that migration from rural to urban mostly takes place to get out of poverty. In other words, poverty emerges as a factor that accelerates migration. With the scarcity of job opportunities in the city and the increase in migration rate; Most of the time, immigrants are exposed to low wage, flexible and insecure conditions in the city. This situation reproduces the state of being poor. Therefore, the identity of immigrants who lose their rights and move away from the sense of equal citizenship will be revealed besides being poor. From this point on, psychological processes related to how immigrants are perceived by society or how they perceive themselves in society emerge. As these psychological processes, we can say; violence, social exclusion, gender discrimination, and prejudice experienced by immigrants. Although these arguments may seem like an outcome of immigration; Since it includes perceptions of both being poor and immigrant, it also points to psychological processes. Here the question of social psychology "what can I do to reduce poverty"; focusing on how immigrants evaluate themselves in their relationship with the local population; It emphasizes the principle of "equal citizenship" in terms of group belonging. This goal can be achieved through multidisciplinary studies to be carried out with local governments, media organizations, and social communication networks.

As we mentioned before, it is necessary to include multiple dimensions and different contexts such as power relations, inequality of opportunity, migration, gender perceptions, family relations, cultural codes, and historical background of the geography in which people live. For example, the migration from rural life to the city, or from one country to the other, especially due to compulsory reasons, may cause to decrease in economic and social resources. And also, social psychology can suggest effective ways for how rural and urban poverty is reflected in intergroup relations given the fact that disadvantaged situations experienced by certain groups, and for how to support structural steps taken to improve the lives of groups affected by poverty [92]. This initiative of social psychology may be effective in the necessity of equal living conditions for all groups. Discussing the dynamics that lead to the perpetuation of economic inequality and poverty with different arguments will lead to studies that allow the interaction of political scientists and psychologists [56]. Similarly, it would be more inclusive to examine poverty as a historical phenomenon (with ideological, psychological, and symbolic aspects). So, it can enable us to focus on the arguments of the capitalist system that are decisive in identity construction [105]. Thus, examining different contexts and representations can prevent the limitations of a research process aimed at testing only hypotheses [87, 106–108]. These multidimensional approaches and analyzes can help reveal potential ideas that can contribute to understanding poverty, preventing and ending it as a pathological phenomenon. So how will it help? The answer to this question will also be the answer to the second question of this study (what role does the proposed integrative approach to poverty analysis play in ending poverty and how is this approach set up?). The content of this analytical framework is shown in **Figure 2**.

According to **Figure 2**; integrative social psychological analysis can help understanding and alleviating poverty in three ways: (1) by including arguments and variables related to psychological and contextual processes in the analysis of poverty, (2) using both empirical (quantitative) research methods that reveal the causality, cause and effect relationships and possible effects of poverty and qualitative research methods that will reveal contextual relationships between arguments, (3) by making macro evaluations of cause-effect and context-specific results, making them applicable in interdisciplinary studies. The combined use of both qualitative and quantitative research methods in poverty studies conducted with a social psychological perspective can provide potential answers to the question of "what can be done to reduce poverty?". The information obtained through this analytical framework can be used in local governments that have responsibility for reducing poverty, in trade union activities that will reinforce the principle of equal citizenship, in migration centers, in media/communication, and some social/political responsibility projects. Undoubtedly, this process can strengthen the cooperation of social psychology with different disciplines and contribute to poverty reduction practices.

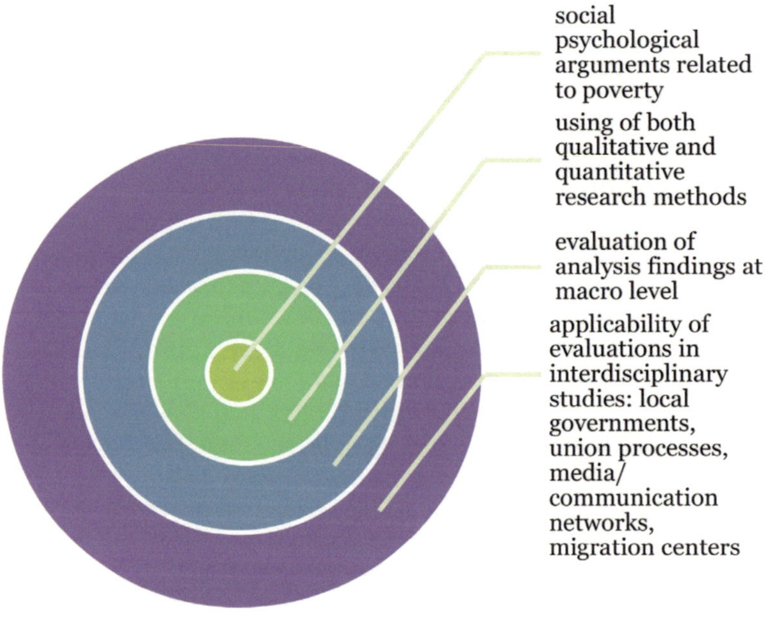

Figure 2.
The key location/role of social psychological analysis in contributing to poverty reduction.

Author details

Filiz Çömez Polat
Psychosocial Department, Credit and Dormitories Agency, The Republic of Turkey Ministry of Youth and Sports, Adana, Turkey

*Address all correspondence to: filiz.ank@gmail.com

References

[1] Leba, R. The importance of the nation-state and the future of the social state in the era of globalization. The Journal of Mevzuat. 2001. 4 (44).

[2] Acıkgoz, R. & Yusufoglu, R. Ö. The phenomenon of poverty and social repercussions in Turkey. Journal of the Human and Social Science Researches. 2012. 1 (1): 76-117.

[3] Allcock, P. Understanding poverty. MacMillanPress; 1997.

[4] Awad, Y. & İsraeli, N. Poverty and income inequality: An international comparison. Available from: http://www.lisproject.org/publications/liswps/166.pdf#search=%22poverty%20and%20income%20inequality. 2010. [Accessed: 09.09.2020]

[5] Hulme, D. & Shepherd, A. Conceptualizing chronic poverty. World Development. 2003. 3: 403-423.

[6] Miller, S. M. The American lower classes: A typological approach. Social Research. 1992. 31 (1): 1-22. Available from www.jstor.org/stable/40969713. [Accessed: 05.08.2020]

[7] Platt L. Poverty studies and social research. In: Holmwood J., Scott J., editors. The Palgrave Handbook of Sociology in Britain. London: Palgrave Macmillan; 2014.

[8] Suğur, N., Suğur, S., Çetin, O., Savran, T. ve Akarcay, E. A research on poverty perceptions of the poor working in the service sector. Is-Guc: The Journal of Industrial Relations & Human Resources. 2008. 10 (4): 1-29.

[9] Townsend, P. Measuring poverty. The British Journal of Sociology. 1954. 5(2): 130-137.

[10] Marshall, G. Sociology dictionary (Translate: Osman Akınhay & Derya Komurcu). İstanbul: Journal of Science and Art Publishing; 1999.

[11] World Bank [Internet]. 2005. Poverty manual. Avaliable from (siteresources.worldbank.org/PGLP/Resources/PMch1.pdf) [Accessed: 16.04.2020]

[12] Rahnema. A world where misery drives out poverty. (Translation: Sule Unsaldı). Ankara: Ozgur University Publications; 2009.

[13] Jensen, E. Teaching with poverty in mind: what being poor does to kids' brains and what schools can do about it. Alexandria, Va: ASCD; 2009.

[14] Ataguba, J.E.O., Ichoku, H.E. & Fonta, W.M. Multidimensional poverty assessment: applying the capability approach. International Journal of Social Economics. 2013. 40 (4): 331-354.

[15] Oktik, N. Conceptual and theoretical approaches to the phenomenon of poverty. In A. D. Sayıcı, editor. Poverty studies in Turkey. İzmir: Yakın Publications; 2008, p. 21-57.

[16] Yüksel, H. General overview on poverty: The sample of OECD countries. Journal of Cankırı Karatekin Univesity-Faculty of Economics and Administrative Sciences. 2014. 4(1): 341-358.

[17] UNDP, Human Development Report. New York: Oxford University Press; 1997, p. 15-16.

[18] Corazzini, L., Esposito, L., & Majorano, F. Exploring the absolutist versus relativist perception of poverty using a cross-country questionnaire survey. Journal of Economic Psychology. 2011. 32: 273-283.

[19] Foster, J. E. Absolute versus relative poverty. American Economic Review. 1998. 88: 335-341.

[20] Yongmie, N. J. Psycho-social dimensions of poverty: When poverty becomes shameful. Critical Social Policy. 2013. 33: 514-531.

[21] Langmore, J. Reducing poverty: The implications of the 1995 Copenhagen Agreement for research on poverty. In D. Gordon, P. Townsend, editors. Breadline Europe: The measurement of poverty. London: Policy Press; 2000, p. 35-47.

[22] Giddens, A. Sociology (Ed. Cemal Guzel). Ankara: Ayrac Publishing; 2005.

[23] Toffler, A.& Toffler, H. Revolutionary wealth. Currency/ Doubleday Publishing; 2006.

[24] TUIK Report:poverty limit. [Internet]. 2012. Available from http://www.tuik.gov.tr/MetaVeri.do?tb_id=23&_id=7. [Accessed: 15.10.2012]

[25] Jones, C., Novak, T. Poverty, welfare and the disciplinary: State of welfare. Psychology Press; 1999.

[26] Lister, R. Poverty. USA: Polity Press Publication; 2004.

[27] Tomlinson, Tomlinson, M., Walker, R., & Williams, G. The relationship between poverty and childhood wellbeing in Great Britain. Barnet Papers in Social Research. Oxford: Department of Social Policy and Social Work, 2008.

[28] Alkier, S., Kanagaratnam, U. & Suppa, N. The global multidimensional poverty index (MPI) 2019: OPHI MPI Methodological Note 47. Oxford Poverty and Human Development Initiative. University of Oxford; 2019.

[29] Beken, H. Conceptualization of poverty [thesis]. University of Marmara; 2006.

[30] Castañeda, A., Doan, D., Newhouse, D., Nguyen, M. C., Uematsu, H., Azevedo, J. P. Policy research paper. World Bank Group. 7844: 2016.

[31] Lewis, H. The culture of poverty? What does it matter? Winter, J. A. (editor). The Poor: A culture of poverty or a poverty of culture? William B. Everdmans Publishing Company, Michingan: Grand Rapids; 1971.

[32] O'Brian, R. Culture of poverty. In Odekaon, M., editor. Encyclopedia of world poverty. Sage Publications, USA; 2006, p. 222-224.

[33] Lewis, O. La Vida (Translate: Vahit Celikbas). İstanbul: E Publishing; 1965.

[34] Akfırat, S.,Çömez-Polat, F., Yetim, Ü. How the poor deal with their own poverty: A social psychological analysis from the social identity perspective. Social Indicators Research. 2016. 127 (1): 413-433.

[35] Carr, S. C. & Bandawe, C. R. Psychology applied to poverty. In Martin, P., Cheung, F., Kyrios, M., Littefield, L., Knowles, M., Prieto, J. M. & Overmier, J. B., editors. The International Association of Applied Psychology (IAAP) handbook of applied psychology Brisbane: Wiley-Blackwell; 2011, p. 639-662.

[36] Brown, C. & Madge, N. Despite the welfare state. Heinemann EB; 1982.

[37] Heaven, C. L. The perceived causal structure of poverty: A network analysis approach. British Journal of Social Psychology. 1994. 33: 259-271.

[38] Birdsall, N. & Homovdi, A. Commodity dependence, trade, and growth: when openness is not enough. Working Paper7. Center for Global Development: Washington, DC; 2002.

[39] Bullock, H. E. & Waugh, I. M. Beliefs about poverty and opportunity among Mexican immigrant

farmworkers. Journal of Applied Social Psychology. 2005. 35: 1132-1149.

[40] Cozzarelli, C., Wilkinson, A. V., & Tagler, M. J. Attitudes toward the poor and attributions for poverty. Journal of Social Issues. 2001. 57: 207-227.

[41] Furnham, A. Poverty and wealth. In Carr, s. C. & Sloan, T.S., editors., Poverty and psychology: From global perspective to local practice. New York: Kluwer Academic/Plenum Publishers; 2003, p. 163-183.

[42] Harvey, D. L. & Reed, M. The culture of poverty: An ideological analyses. Sociological Perspective. 1996. 34 (4): 465-495.

[43] Jordon, G. The causes of poverty culture vs structural: can there be a synthesis? Spring Publishing; 2004.

[44] Muncer, S. & Gillen, K. The perceived causes of poverty: a question of politics. Paper presented at Annual Conference of the British Psychological Society. University of Warwick: UK; 1995.

[45] Townsend, P. Poverty in the United Kingdom. Penguin Publications; 1978.

[46] Walker, R. Poverty dynamics. Avebury: Aldershot; 1994.

[47] Solak, N & Göregenli, M. Development and evaluation of the psychometric properties of the attributions for poverty scale. Turkish Psychological Articles. 2009. 12: 72-89.

[48] Hine, D. W., & Montiel, C. J. Poverty in developing nations: Cultural attributional analysis. European Journal of Social Psychology. 1999. 29(7): 943-959.

[49] Feagin, J. R. Poverty: we still believe that God helps those who help themselves. Psychology Today. 1972. 6: 101-129.

[50] Bullock, H.E. From the frontlines of welfare reform: An analysis of social worker and welfare recipient attitudes. Journal of Social Psychology. 2004. 144: 571-588.

[51] Harper, D. J. Poverty and discourse. In Carr, S. T. & Sloan, T. S., editors. International and cultural psychology series. Poverty and psychology: From global perspective to local practice. Kluwer Academic/Plenum Publishers; 2003, p. 185-203.

[52] Göregenli, M. Reflections on fact-value relationship in social sciences based on social psychology. Society and Science. 2003. 97: 234-246.

[53] Reid, P. T. Poor women in psychological research: Shut up and shut out. Psychology of Women Quarterly. 1993. 17: 133-150.

[54] Lemieux, A. F. ve Pratto, F. Poverty and prejudice. In Carr, S. and Sloan, editors. Poverty and psychology: From global perspective to local practice. New York: Kluwer Academic Publishers; 2003, p. 147-161.

[55] Tajfel, H., & Turner, J. C. The social identity theory of intergroup behavior. In Worchel, S. & Austin, W. G., editors. Psychology of intergroup relations. Chicago: Nelson-Hallnel; 1986, p. 7-24.

[56] Jetten, J. & Peter, K. Putting a social psychological spotlight on economic inequality. In Jetten, J. & Peter, K., editors. The social psychology of inequality. Springer International Publishing; 2019, p. 1-18.

[57] Bratanova, B., Summers, J., Liv, S. & Vouclair, C. M. Rising tide lifts some boats but leaves many others behind: the harms of inequality induced status seeking and the remadial effects of employce ownership. In Jetten, J. & Peter, K., editors. The social psychology of inequality Springer International Publishing; 2019, p. 83-102.

[58] Cheung, F. & Lucas, R. F. Income inequality is associated with stronger social comparison effecs: the effect of relative income on life satisfaction. Journal of Personality and Social Psychology. 2016. 110 (2): 332-341.

[59] Walasek, L. & Brown, G. Income inequality and social status: the social rank and material rank hypotheses. In Jetten, J. & Peter, K., editors. The social psychology of inequality Springer International Publishing; 2019, p. 260-275.

[60] Ximenes, V, M., Cidade, E. C., Silva, G. Psychology research in the poverty context: what for and whom? In Ximenes, M. V., Moura, Jr. J.J.F., Cidade, E., Nepomuceno, B., editors. Psychosocial implications of poverty: Diversities and resistances Springer Nature Switzerland AG; 2019, p. 3-16.

[61] Guzzo, R. S. Social inequality and psychology: perspective for debate on poverty. In Ximenes, M. V., Moura, Jr. J.J.F., Cidade, E., Nepomuceno, B., editors. Psychosocial implications of poverty: Diversities and resistance. Springer Nature Switzerland AG; 2019, p. 37-45.

[62] Okoroji, C., Gleibs, I. H. & Jovchelovitch, S. Elite stigmatization of the unemployed: the association between framing and public attitudes. British Journal of Psychology. 2020. Available from www.onlinelibrarywiley.com/doi/epdf/10111/bjop.12450. [Accessed: 10.09.2020]

[63] Aguilar, G. S & Sumner, A. Who are the world's poor? A new profile of global multidimensional poverty. Working Paper, 2019. Available from https://www.cgdev.org/sites/default/files/who-are-worlds-poor-new-profile-global-multidimensional-poverty.pdf . [Accessed from: 22.09.2020]

[64] Alkier, S., Nogales, R., Quinn, N. N. & Suppa, N. On track or not? Projecting the global multidimensional poverty index. OPHI Research in Progress 58a. Oxford Poverty and Human Development Initiative. University of Oxford; 2020.

[65] Lewis, O. The culture of poverty. [Internet]. 1966. Available from www.lenguaix.pbworks.com/f/Culture+of+Poverty.pdf . [Accessed: 07.09.2020]

[66] Bakker, B. N. Personality traits, income and economic ideology. Journal of Political Psychology. 2016. 38 (6): 1025-1041.

[67] Hart, D., Atkins, R. & Matsuba, M. K. The association of neighborhood poverty with personality change in childhood. Journal of Personality and Social Psychology. 2008. 94: 1048-1061.

[68] Sawhill, I. V. The behavioral aspects of poverty. [Internet]. 2003. Available from www.edu/articles/the-behavioral-aspects-of-poverty. [Accessed: 06.09.2020]

[69] Diener, E. & Biswas-Diener, R. Will money increase subjectivity well-being? Social Indicators Research. 2002. 57 (2): 119-169.

[70] Elliott, I. Poverty and mental health: A review to inform the Joseph Rowntree Foundations anti-poverty strategy. London: Mental Health Foundation; 2016.

[71] Fell, B. & Hewstone, M. Psychological perspectives on poverty. JRF Report. 2015. Available from https://www.jrf.org.uk/report/psychological-perspectives-poverty. [Accessed: 16.10.2020]

[72] Frankenhuis, W. E. & Nettler, D. The strengths of people in poverty. Current Directions in Psychological Science. 2020. 29 (1): 16-21.

[73] Funk, M, Drew, N. & Knapp, M. Mental health, poverty and

development. Journal of Public Mental Health. 2012. 11 (4): 166-185.

[74] Lever, J.P.L., Pimnol, N.L.& Uralde, J. H. Poverty, psychological resources and subjective well-being. Social Indicators Research. 2005. 73: 375-408.

[75] Mullainathan, S. & Shafir, E. Scarcity: Why having too little means so much. Journal of Human Behaviour in the Social. 2013. 25 (3): 284-286.

[76] Rojas, M. Experienced poverty and income poverty in Mexico: A subjective well-being approach. World Development. 2008. 36: 1078-1093.

[77] Yoshikawa, H.,Aber, L.& BeardsleeW. The effects of poverty on the mental, emotional and behavioral health of children and youth implications for prevention. American Psychologist. 2012. 67 (4): 272-284.

[78] Clark, A., D'Ambrosio, C., Ghislendi, S. Poverty and well-being: panel evidence from Germany. Society for the Study of Economic Inequality Working Papers. 2013. Available from www.ecineq.org. [Accessed: 05.08.2020]

[79] McGillivray, M. Inequality, poverty and well-being. In M. McGillavray, editor. Inequality, poverty and wellbeing. Palgrave Macmilla UK; 2006.

[80] Moussa-Simona, J. The subjective well-being of those vulnerable to poverty in Switzerland. Journal of Happiness Studies. 2019. 21: 1561-1580.

[81] Pift, P. K., Moscowitz, P. J. Wealth, poverty and happiness: social class is differentially associated with positive emotions. Emotion. 2018. 18 (6): 902-905.

[82] Mowat, J., G. Exploring the impact of social inequality and poverty on the mental health, well-being and attainment of children and young people in Scotland. SAGE Journals. 2018. 22 (3): 204-223.

[83] Dao, M.Q. Human capital, poverty, and income distribution in developing countries. Journal of Economic Studies. 2008. 35 (4): 94-303.

[84] Domfeh, K.A. & Bawole, J.N. Localising and sustaining poverty reduction: Experiences from Ghana. Management of Environmental Quality: An International Journal. 2009. 20 (5): 490-505.

[85] Houshofer, J. Is there a psychological poverty trap? [Internet]. 2019. Available from www.princeton.edu/houshofer-psychological-trap-2019-pdf. [Accessed: 14.09.2020]

[86] Kayaoğlu, A. Prejudice against the poor: a way of depoliticizing poverty. International for Theoretical Psychology Biennial Meeting, Theoretical Psychology beyond borders: transdisciplinary and internationalization, June 18-22, Toronto., 2007.

[87] O'Connor, A. Poverty knowledge: social science, social policy and the poor in twentieth-century US history. Princeton and Oxford: Princeton University Press; 2001.

[88] Carr, S. C. Anti-poverty psychology. In Marcella, A. C., editor. International and cultural psychology. Newyork: Springer; 2012.

[89] Harper, D. J. Accounting for poverty.: from attribution to discourse. Journal of Community & Applied Social Psychology. 1996. 6: 249-265.

[90] Connoly, K. Psychology and poverty. Bulletin of the British Psychological Society. 1982. 35: 1-9.

[91] Carr, S. C., & Sloan, T. S. (Eds.). (2003). International and cultural psychology series. Poverty and psychology: From global perspective to local practice. Kluwer Academic/ Plenum Publishers; 2003.Available

from: https://doi.org/10.1007/978-1-4615-0029-2. [Accessed: 04.09.2020]

[92] Novak, T. Rethinking poverty. Journal of Critical Social Policy. 1995. 15: 58-74.

[93] Perez, A., Fuertez, F., Arias, R. An explanatory model of poverty from the perspective of social psychology and human rights. The Spanish Journal of Psychology. 2015.

[94] Edwards, D. ve Potter, J. Discursive Psychology, London. 1992.

[95] Wetherell, M. Themes in discourse research: The case of Diana. M. Wetherell; S. Taylor; Yates, S.(eds) Discourse theory and practice: A Reader, s/14-28, London: Sage Publication. 2001.

[96] Harré, R. Singular Self. London: Sage. 1998

[97] Fairclough, Norman. Critical discourse analysis. Marges Linguistiques, 2005, 9: 76-94

[98] Van Dijk, Teun A. Society and discourse: How social contexts influence text and talk. Cambridge: Cambridge University Press. 2009b.

[99] Parker, I. Revolution in psychology: Alıneation to emancipation. Pluto Press: London. 2007.

[100] Arkonaç, S.Psikolojide söz ve anlam analizi. Istanbul: Ayrıntı Publication. 2014.

[101] Golding, P. & Middleton, S. Images of welfare: Press and public attitudes to poverty. Oxford: Martin Robertson. 1982.

[102] Topçuğlu, A., Aksan, G. & Alptekin, D. Poverty and woman. İstanbul: Ayrıntı Publication. 2016.

[103] ECLAC Report. Economic comission for Latin America and Carribbean (ECLAC) understanding poverty from a gender perspective. 2004. www.repositorio.cepal.org/bitstream/handle/11362/5926/1S04646.on.pdf

[104] Chant, S. Fairness & equality. Available from: www.blogs/ıse.ac.uk. politics andpolicy/gender/poverty/links. 2011. [Accesed: 09.06.2020]

[105] Estanislau, M. A. & Ximenes, V. M. Experiences of humiliation and shame: A psychological analysis in contexts of poverty. In Jetten, J. & Peter, K., editors. The Social psychology of inequality. Springer International Publishing; 2019, p. 260-275.

[106] Ximenes, M. V., Maura, Jr. J.F., Cidade, E. C. & Nepomuceno, B.B. (Eds). Psychosocial implications of poverty: diversities and resistances. Springer Nature Switzerland AG; 2019.

[107] Accorssi, A. & Scarpano, H. Social representations of poverty. In Ximenes, M. V., Moura, Jr. J.J.F., Cidade, E.& Nepomuceno, B., editors. Psychosocial implications of poverty: diversities and resistances. Switzerland AG: Springer Nature; 2019, p.17-35.

[108] Kayaoğlu, A. Psychology of poverty or poverty of psychology: Criticism of psychological poverty approaches. The Journal of Theory and Research. 2008. 27: 99-126.

Chapter 8

Zambia's Poorest Progressively Left Behind: Well-Being Denied

Brendan P. Carmody

Abstract

After Independence in 1964, the government of Zambia set out to fashion a national of equals. In this, the school was seen to be a key strategy along the lines of the modernisation route to development. Initially, this seemed to be well directed but within a short time it was evident that this mode of schooling was elitist, promoting division between 'haves' and 'have-nots.' Today, the country is greatly divided between those who are well-off and those who are not. This article traces the path to this outcome historically.

Keywords: Zambia, equity, school, modernization, marginalization, educational reform, equality of access, opportunity structure

1. Introduction

In the years following Independence in 1964, Zambia, like many African states, viewed education to be pivotal to its development as a nation. This belief in the power of school was partly grounded in what is known as the modernization approach which emphasizes investment in the formation of labour capital [1]. The political leaders were concerned with economic progress and the need to build an inclusive nation [2].

As this mode of national development has emerged, we find that in 2013 a Catholic secondary school in Lusaka's Matero township, a densely populated low-income section of the city, had approximately 10 percent of its students from the local district. This was because the local children did not reach the school's Grade VII qualifying grade [3]. As a result, the school, like many other private or semi-private schools, had a preponderance of its students from outside the immediate surroundings.

Matero Boys is grant-aided which means that it follows government direction and is also Church sponsored. It thus follows government practice of admitting those who reach a certain academic standard in the belief that this meritocratic way of proceeding is equitable and fair in avoiding marginalization and providing equal opportunity to all [4]. Yet, this mode of procedure appears to work against one of the Catholic school's prime purposes—inclusion of those at the margins. To better appreciate this paradoxical situation, we turn to a review of its setting.

2. Context

As a Catholic school, Matero boys is part of a long tradition that heralds social justice which includes concern for the poorest. The first Catholic missionaries generally set up outposts where missionaries had outreach to the poor and were oftentimes accused of giving handouts [5]. Similarly, it is true that in later times such missionaries were branded as instruments of colonialism in so far as they are said to have cooperated with the British colonial state. A significant aspect of this emerged when, by adopting the school as a means of evangelization, the colonial government became more directive. At that point in the late 1920s, the Catholic school, as others, was faced with a dilemma. It could continue largely outside government jurisdiction as a church school or it could become part of the colonial state system.

Missionaries found themselves on both sides of this issue but with the visit of Monsignor Arthur Hinsley, the voice of Rome, Catholic missionaries were told to place their schools within the state framework [6]. For the most part, they did this even if sometimes reluctantly. In the long term, this proved to be a good means of outreach in so far as it promised people from the remotest areas escape from the village and the opportunity to find wage labour in the developing mines and towns. Attending school was a means for Northern Rhodesians (Zambians after 1964) to become what has been called the fortunate few [7]. What is evident is that the early missionaries directed their efforts at assisting the poor and, given the climate of the time, they could be seen to be weakly aware of the political implications of their activities one of which included the price of becoming part of the colonial state system.

After a Church Council called Vatican II ending in 1965, the Church adopted a more political approach with an emphasis on social justice [8]. It stressed individual human rights but extended this to what it called the common good where each person's participation in the general welfare is highlighted [9]. This ideal was elucidated principally in 1968 through a papal document called *Populorum Progressio* and formed a key aspect of the Latin American bishops' conference in Medellin in 1968 [10]. It meant that missionaries began to be conscious of the political dimension of their schools [11].

This took place in the years after 1965 when Zambia was striving to establish itself as a newly Independent state and, as already indicated, it placed a heavy emphasis on education and, under the leadership of President Kaunda, the ideal of equity was fore-grounded. One might conjecture that this meant support for the promotion of social justice and the ideal that everyone would share equitably in the new nation's development. In that respect, the poorest seemed to have equal opportunity. What was new within this viewpoint, from the point of view of the Catholic Church, was that liberation of the poorest assumed a social structural or political framework. While the old system of assisting individuals to gain uplift remained, the church began to focus on social structures and their capacity to promote or impede social justice. In this way of thinking it was argued that there was a need to contribute towards building a just social order [12]. More specifically, a document called *The Catholic School* notes:

> *Since it is motivated by the Christian ideal, the Catholic school is particularly sensitive to the call from every part of the world for a more just society, and it tries to make its contribution towards it. It does not stop at the courageous teaching of the demands of justice even in the face of local opposition, but it tries to put these demands into practice in its own community in the daily life of the school [13].*

The same document affirmed that, first and foremost, the church offers its educational service to the poor and if the church turns its attention exclusively to those who are wealthier it would be contributing to their privileged position and would thereby favour the development of a society that is unjust.

In this context of commitment to the poorest as developed in terms of the common good, we have the Matero Boys situation where the local poorest are excluded, not because they are unable to pay as was true elsewhere [14], but because they failed to meet government-set academic criteria for entry. One could argue that what Edward Berman spoke about, when he charged missionaries of subordinating their mission to government aims, had come to pass [15]. However, it could also be argued that this was not the case but that the church under the authority of the Zambian Ministry of Education which is now called Ministry of Education, Science, Vocational Training and Early Education (MESVTEE) the merit-based educational system provides an avenue towards equity and social justice and thus avoids marginalization of the poorest [16].

What follows argues that this claim is false but was uncritically accepted as true by the Catholic Church and more widely. It is a historical approach illustrating how, despite government intentions to create a nation that would not marginalize, the Zambian school system became a pivotal instrument of progressively excluding large sectors of society from the fruits of economic development which meant decreasing access to formal employment and the well-being that it promised.

The discussion emerges from secondary sources--published work, books, journals, educational reports on reforms, adjustments to World Bank demands, undergirded by the author's long-time experience in the country as a teacher, administrator, and researcher. It engages with such issues as the ideal of justice, opportunity structure, upward mobility, class formation, educational reform, education as reproductive of the status quo as it develops the the notion of marginalization. This speaks of social groups especially the poor in rural areas and densely parts of towns or cities as well as subgroups whose voices were weakly heard—girls, orphans, and those with special needs. As will be seen, the process of marinalization gains momentum when in the mid 1970s a new-found social elite gain control of the education system and strive to ensure that access to school maintains and reproduces its privileged position as the majority are left out.

3. The evolution of Zambia's education System

On gaining Independence in 1964 the new Zambian government had an extremely limited pool of educated labour. Out of a population of about four million only 110,000 had received six years of schooling and of these only fifty-eight percent had completed full primary school. Fourteen percent had passed the two-year junior secondary course as 961 had completed the Cambridge School Certificate [17]. In this setting, government realized that education was a major priority so that it could place its heavily marginalized people in positions of responsibility in the new state.

At the same time, the government lost no time in assuming almost total control of the education system through an Education Act in 1966. Subsequently, its Ministry of Education quickly expanded access to schooling so as to provide universal primary education for every Zambian, which had been a long-term ideal [18]. Given the challenge of creating a nation-state, government also saw schooling as a means towards national unity and prosperity for all. However, within that perspective, the President was concerned to develop a nation where there would be little division between 'haves' and 'have-nots' [19]. In its egalitarian concern, the Ministry of Education abolished school fees so that schooling would be open to all unlike what had been the case during colonialism.

4. Equity and prosperity through modernization

In pursuing this aim of promoting widespread education for prosperity and inclusion, government adopted what, at the time was seen to be the best or only route, which was seen to be that of modernization [20]. This theory had been popularized in the 1950s and 60s to explain the relative under-development of Latin America, Africa, and Asia. It equated their current stage of under-development to an earlier historical period of the developed nations. It thereby assumed that development was unilinear consisting of a sequence of stages. One of its earliest proponents was Walter Rostow who spoke of the traditional, pre-condition, and take off stages [21].

Among the pivotal preconditions for the so-called take off, Rostow identified the development of natural science and technology and the values that accompany them. This came to mean that academic schooling was seen to be a crucial ingredient. Through the school, children would learn the tools of becoming modern. A key element of this theory would be that the nation-state. Developing countries could pursue a path to their development even if they might helpfully seek advice and assistance from developed countries. Subsequent development of Rostow's thesis occurred with articulation in 1961 of what was called the human capital approach where education came to be seen as an important investment which would lead to national prosperity [22]. This theory emphasized development of urban modern industrial centres which would then spread employment and prosperity to the whole population.

With this international framework for development in view, Zambia invested heavily in schooling, patterned on the educational systems of Europe with the hope that it would lead to widespread prosperity at the national level. It was founded in an understanding that school had a direct impact on producing a developed nation which would mean widespread, if not full, employment of those educated. In the Zambian context, it meant that government introduced what was a conventionally academic approach to school and saw success in the state academic examinations as perhaps the best and fairest means to national development in so far as it offered equality of access to all though free schools.

As a result, between 1964 and 1970, the number of children in primary schools increased dramatically as it did also at secondary as well as teacher and university education [23]. This surge of enrollment continued as the economy was buoyant and appeared to promise widespread schooling and opportunity to all, which accorded well with the government's desire to create a nation of equals where even the poorest child in the far off regions of the country would not be marginalized but would have equal chance to succeed as those in the cities coming from well-to-do families. In these early years, where formal employment was abundant for schooled people at primary level and beyond, the system was widely welcomed and enabled many of the poor to move up the social ladder.

5. The centre did not hold

Within a few years however this pattern of providing universal schooling and the opportunities that accompanied it began to show signs of break-down. By 1969, despite the promise of universal access to primary school, 33 percent of the seven-year old children were not in school and many of those who completed their primary schooling could not find places in secondary schools [24]. The ideal of universal primary schooling and wholesale employment in the formal sector were in question.

In subsequent years (1970-1975), the situation deteriorated with increasing numbers being excluded from the system at primary, secondary, and tertiary levels in part because the government could no longer afford to provide the kind of universal access which it had originally promised. This needs to be seen particularly in light of the adverse economic situation for Zambia in the 1970s when the price of its main market product—copper—fell dramatically. In the situation of a growing squeeze on revenue and an increasing limit of access to school, by 1975 only 49 percent of the 7-14 year olds were in school.

6. Modernization under short-term review

With awareness of this fast-growing problem of over-emphasis on academic schooling and its failure to deliver equal opportunity and social inclusion in the early 1970s, the government sought an alternative route to development which questioned the modernization school model along socialist lines. The President noted the growing economic and social gap between the urban and rural population as well as the fact that new-found wealth was concentrated in the hands of a small but powerful group where the masses were increasingly marginalized [25].

At the same time, dependency theorists argued against a linear perspective on national development and spoke of core and periphery dimensions of such development within the capitalist order [26]. At the periphery where developing nations were located, development depended principally on what happened in the developed nations at the core. These nations in turn depended on the periphery for their own development and so economic development at the margins was highly dependent, resembling what had taken place in colonial times. Dependency theorists advocated cutting links with the modernization approach and promoting self-reliance. This was already occurring in places like Tanzania and Cuba. Efforts had already been made to diversify the curriculum along these lines but they seemed to be inadequate [27].

It is therefore not so astonishing that in 1973, the President called for a major review of the education system which resulted in a widespread survey, consultation, and a subsequent proposal, *Education for Development* [28]. It spoke of equity and the need to provide a system that did not favour a minority of the population by preparing an elite for high-status and leadership positions. Though there was appreciation for what the then current system offered in terms of social mobility for the less well-off, it pointed to the growing tendency to become socially reproductive. In that way it enhanced the position of those in power enabling them to maintain their privilege. It was recognized that continuation of the then current education system would result in shrinkage of the opportunity structure for the poorest. In addition, *Education for Development* questioned the value of schools that were oriented to passing exams with little or no consideration of their wider national economic and industrial roles. It likened the system to a train that travels on a single track bound for one destination ejecting most of the passengers on the way, keeping a small minority [29]. It was nonetheless acknowledged that changing the educational system in itself was insufficient; there was need to transform the socio-economic setting [30]. This signaled anxiety and resistance for those already benefitting from the system.

Though the proposal was debated at some length, it was swiftly rejected in favour of essentially maintaining the then current system but including what might be identified as cosmetic reforms in *Educational Reform* [31]. The revised model focused on capacity building and emphasized education as an instrument for personal and national development. The system took on additional features including keeping an eye on rural development and self-reliance inspired by what appeared to be happening in places like Cuba and Tanzania. By keeping this ideal of self-reliance in the background, it was hoped that national development could be better balanced between what was happening in the urban and rural settings and as a consequence that employment would not be so heavily focused on academic merit. It was moreover seen to be a better way to avoid creating a nation with 'haves' linked to jobs in the town and 'have-nots' in the rural areas.

As the country emerged from the so-called reforms in 1977, it was clear that control of the system was passing into the hands of what had developed as an elite who had become politically powerful. It favoured the modernization approach to development in its academically selective process even though this meant ever increasing numbers who would be marginalized by it. While, theoretically, the system was still free and open to all, because of its academic and Western-style curriculum including English as the medium of instruction, it favoured those who had become part of the growing elite, becoming reproductive of their status and less disposed to upward mobility for the many at the margins [32].

What resulted was a continuation of the system as it was but it kept in view the government's commitment to the promotion of equity in terms of a widespread access to primary schooling. Though this appeared to manifest concern for the so-called marginalized masses, it did not greatly impact the academically selective system which continued to favour those who were part of the growing elite [33]. In addition, because of government's debt, fees were introduced a few years later at different levels, which more severely impacted the poor.

With the introduction of fees at various points of the system, the Catholic Church, among others, pleaded on behalf of the marginalized sections of society and began to provide grants and bursaries. It had earlier praised the momentum of the first education reform proposal, *Education for Development,* for its emphasis on including the weaker elements of society and in general came to find itself at odds with the elitist system that had now emerged. It did not openly advocate for radical review or take major steps against what was taking place. This may indeed confirm Berman, in seeing the church subordinating its mission, but it probably makes some sense in so far as the church had to thread a tight line as the state became more authoritarian and intolerant of alternative viewpoints [34].

7. Modernization amended

Meanwhile, the education system continued to be informed by a human capital outlook leading to an elitist status for a minority while the political rhetoric spoke in terms of production units and local empowerment. By 1980, there were 493,000 employed in the formal sector of the economy which represented about 27 percent of the working-age sector. Already, 14 percent of the unemployed had some secondary schooling with most from the earlier drop-out points Grade 4 and Grade 7. Progression to Grade 8 pivoted at about 23 percent which meant that large numbers were being forced to leave school with little prospect of formal employment. This concern of relating school with access to jobs had been a crucial issue in the so-called reform movement but little had been done beyond discussion [35]. The curriculum had been designed to secure entry to school and to lead to formal employment. This was happening less and less with more and more children being marginalized. Linear expansion of the system was not sufficient [36].

Although there were piecemeal attempts to implement the so-called education reform, no comprehensive approach took place till, at the instigation of the World Bank, a major survey was undertaken and a report appeared in 1986 known as the *Educational Reform Implementation Project* (ERIP) [37]. This document focused on the need for equity in educational development and was seen to be best approached by according priority to primary schooling. It was seen in the light of employment opportunities which left many without the possibility of formal employment. The concern became: how could the school system be revamped to assist the increasing numbers of those who were being marginalized which progressively meant the poorest in society? [38].

In response to the World Bank's directives and promise of assistance, ERIP proposed large-scale investment in what had been an initial ideal namely primary schooling for all Zambian children [39]. In so doing, there was also a proposed moratorium on investment in secondary and higher education. At the primary level, it meant expansion of provision which led to the construction of schools and invitation to the local community to help in this project. In many instances, the response of the community was predominantly to construct basic schools (schools that added facilities for Grade 7 and 8). This led to increased enrolment in what would often be rather make-shift schools throughout the country and many of these allowed children to enter the lower secondary school level (basic included Grades 8 and 9 which were lower secondary), adding to what already was a bad situation:

Reports from several parts of the country drew attention to the bad physical condition of school buildings... cracked walls... termite infested... broken or missing doors, windows without glass... leaking water ... blocked toilets [40].

ERIP thus concentrated on how to achieve the long cherished ideal of seven years primary school for every Zambian child, despite a bleak economic climate where government struggled to pay the nation's external debt and was subjected to conditions set by the International Monetary Fund known as Structural Adjustment Programme (SAP). *Educational Reform Implementation Project* considered that by widening the net at the primary school level economic growth would be enhanced. It claimed that returns to investment in primary schooling were greater nationally than at higher levels. Besides, investment per student at this level was hugely less costly than investment than at university level [41].

What was ambiguous was that the report appeared to envisage primary schooling (and less obvioulsy basic schooling) to be the end of the road for most children but that did not fit the long-term understanding that primary school's real value in the minds of children and their parents. They saw it as a stepping stone to Grade 8 and beyond; hence, local community's support for basic schools which not only allowed more primary-aged children to be admitted but enabled most of them to stay to Grade 9. The report paradoxically also envisaged the introduction of fees because of the poor condition of the nation's financial situation, breaking the welfare state system of free schooling that had characterized the nation since Independence and threatening the welfare and access to school for those who were poor [42].

8. Achieving primary education for all

To address the challenge of including all children in quality primary school as a prelude to better economic standing, the new MMD government continued to emphasize self-reliance through production units but after 1991 sought more input from the local community as it further transformed the country into a market-based economy. Under this government, Zambia committed itself to the *World Declaration on Education for All.* Enrolment in primary (Grades 1-7) and basic (Grades 1-9) increased as initiatives to ensure better inclusion of girls, orphans, special needs, and rural children followed as did monitoring of attainment of basic literacy.

Nonetheless, enrolment levels were constrained by the introduction of fees in a climate of widespread unemployment as well as by an increasing lack of confidence in the system to deliver much coveted formal employment as the opportunity structure contracted [43]. Fees disproportionately impacted the poor many of whom not only failed to enroll but after enrolment were likely to drop out. Most parents could not afford to meet the obligatory costs of sending their children to school [44]. By 1998, the national average attendance in primary school was 66 percent of which only 50 percent progressed to Grades 8 and about 20 percent to Grade 10. This represented 61 percent in rural versus 80 percent in urban areas [45]. Not only did this reveal how rural children were marginalized but, despite efforts to assist, those excluded were disproportionately girls, those with special needs, and orphans [46].

However, though the overall impact was that the intake into the primary schools increased, because of government's financial situation and input, many of the schools were of poor quality leaving one wonder about the level of literacy of those who completed at either primary or basic level [47]. These basic schools provided wider access. However, only 64 percent of richer families enrolled in them. Instead, the better endowed opted for private or faith-based schools some of which did not transform their lower secondary schools to become basic. As a result, they had better facilities which promised better quality learning, increasing their chances of what was severely limited, entry to Grade 10 [48].

This overall movement towards primary and in some cases basic education for all became a leading motif within the system under strain. As a result, by 2001, the primary school enrollment reached 1.77 million as against 1.4 million in 1990. This modest increase nonetheless meant that 65 percent equal to 700,000 of seven-year-olds were not in school. Of those who completed primary school, roughly 50 percent proceeded to Grade 8 (because of the basic school movement) and approximately 20 percent to Grade 10 which represented a significant drop-out rate especially at the end of Grade 9.

A key reason for the large out of school population was that, because of fees, the poorest were excluded. Yet, while the overall number gaining primary school education had increased, this did not translate into the fact that they would gain formal employment. What we have instead is a better schooled population within a declining employment rate [49]. Investment in education on a national level had not expanded economic productivity as had been promised and expected. Moreover, in this expansion of provision, as already indicated, the quality of schooling was uneven especially in rural areas, leaving those that completed largely and progressively less qualified in their search for formal employment.

Though basic literacy is to be prized as a human right, the universal primary school movement appears to have done little to enable those with primary or basic schooling to avoid marginalization and climb the educational pyramid especially since investment and expansion at the secondary level and higher level had been somewhat frozen. Yet, clearly that was what most desired in the interest of finding formal employment. It came to mean that more and more young people emerged from basic schools with slimmer and slimmer chances of being selected to go further. The opportunities for entry to Grade 10 were clearly linked to those who had quality schooling, which in rural and poor urban communities was less likely because of deprived facilities. Related to this, the question emerged: what was the economic or social value of these years in school when at the end graduates could not find formal employment? This needs to be seen within the context where about 10 percent of Zambia's employment was then at the formal level [50].

Since the majority of children who entered Grade I were blocked from ascending the ladder to higher secondary school (high school as it was called for some years) and beyond, the age-old question of seeking a different kind of schooling re-emerged. Though numbers in school increased, the problem of formal employment for those who emerged remained, resembling what it had happened in the colonial times. It was the long and fast developing problem of 'educated unemployed' [51]. Juxtaposed to this was the high poverty level ranging at about 80 percent of the population.

As the overall population increased and as the country went through financial struggle, the Ministry of Education sought more community (local and international) support, moving one might say from a welfare state to a market-based economy. In that setting it pressed ahead with the goal of universal primary schooling under the impression that this was the route not only to greater prosperity but to decreased marginalization and more equitable distribution of resources. The decade between 1990 and 2001 thus witnessed increased enrollment but did little for what was the major concern namely formal employment bringing again to focus the question of how appropriate was the school curriculum for job creation [52].

Attention inevitably focused on the nature and role of the Technical Education, Vocational, and Entrepreneurship Authority (TEVETA) which had been set up in the past and provided education more directly linked to employable skills. In 2000, 151 institutions under its control had an overall enrollment of 24,648 students. One might wonder why these settings with promise of some formal and self-employment had not become more attractive. It is true that many were private which entailed fees but perhaps more pivotally academic schooling had been seen for generations to be the pathway to formal and well-paid employment [53]. Thus, getting people interested in this technical mode of schooling proved to be difficult even if it promised to assist students to become productive particularly in the informal sector [54].

In any event, in the light of ERIP, by 2001, there was 1.770,000 million pupils in primary school and the progression rate to Grade 8 had pivoted around 35 percent. This overall increase in the primary and basic school populations resulted in large part because of the growth of basic and latterly community schools [55]. Though both these models of school made a major contribution in reducing the number of out-of-school children largely because they were free, they operated in ways that were rudimentary [56].

As Zambia gained relief from its debt through the Heavily Indebted Poor Countries (HIPC) initiative in 2002, one of its first responses was again to provide free basic schooling in view of achieving universal primary schooling which had been such a long-term issue. This helped. Implementation and interpretation of this free schooling revealed 'hidden' fees as well as increased quantity at the cost of quality. There were too many over-crowded classrooms and schools with shortage of teachers. This was especially true in rural areas and densely populated sectors of cities and towns [57].

Following the re-introduction of the free basic schooling in 2002, enrollments increased though the degree to which the schools were free remained an on-going question. Correlated with this was government's inadequate support of school infrastructural needs [58]. By 2008, enrollments had increased to 2,909,436 at the primary level and 3,290,000 at the basic level [59]. This could clearly be seen as a major step forward in the goal of providing primary schooling for all Zambian children even if it included a low intake rate of 56 percent for the age 7-13 [60]. This pattern of increased enrollment was enhanced in the years following by economic growth in the economy largely because of increased copper sales and greater government investment in schooling.

9. Modernization with new horizons

As the enrollment at the primary and basic levels moved towards the goal of primary schooling for all, it is not surprising that government's attention moved towards expansion of the secondary and higher levels, which had been on hold since the late 1980s in order to support the movement towards universal primary education as the best effort towards equity creation. This shift to post-primary was also prompted by the fact that the workforce grew at an annual average rate of 4.9 percent between 2005 and 2012. Increasingly, employment went to the more educated. Those with no education and those with Grade 7 found it harder to get jobs while those with Grades 8-12 s and university level had a better chance, prompting a perceived need for higher academic credentials.The majority of school leavers were thus marginalized and faced with employment in the informal sector which TEVET supported. Despite government rhetoric however, its investment in TEVET compared poorly with that of other sectors especially the university [61].

When the Patriotic Front (PF) government was elected in 2011, it took steps to include more people at the higher levels of the education system. As part of its approach, it renamed and reframed the educational system, reverting to the older system of speaking of primary school as Grades 1–7, secondary school Grades 8–12 followed by tertiary education. The previous system had been introduced to facilitate the inclusion of Grades 8 and 9. The problem had now shifted to include more pupils in Grades 8-12. Access to secondary school and higher levels of education was seen to be part of the route to achieving the country's middle-income status in the light of Vision 2030. At the same time, government recognized that the dynamic of the current system of education poorly related to the creation of employment and as a result the country still wrestled with high level poverty and marginalization. Would large-scale investment at the higher levels create more employment or would school leavers face the need for higher credentials for roughly the same level of formal employment?

10. Modernization reframed

With dramatic expansion at secondary and higher level enrolment in view, the PF government decided through *Framework 2012* [62] to leave the system fundamentally as it was but to balance the curriculum so that the technical learning might no longer be seen to be inferior [63]. Instead of a major effort at reform of the system as happened in the mid-1970s, it proposed a two-career twin pathway in the school curriculum–academic and technical. This re-emphasis and effort to better include technical education together with a review of English being displaced by local languages at the lower Grades as the medium of instruction could be seen to re-surface the age-old issue of the relevance of the predominant kind of the schooling on offer. In an effort towards greater inclusion and less marginalization, it also opened pre-schools so that head-starts were not monopolized by the better off members of society.

This concern to integrate the different streams of schooling appears to be well directed but to be effective in breaking the age-old bias against technical education, the overall system may need a greater commitment to educate for formal employment and greater backing for TEVET's 275 institutions. Currently, the almost exclusive human capital perspective on social development continues to dominate and to be reproductive of the social order with highly unsatisfactory implications for inclusion of the majority. As, at the time of the so-called education reform in 1976, making this job-oriented learning attractive promises to be a hard battle. In the minds of most, formal employment is linked to academic achievement [64]. In some instances as in the case of university academic staff, this appears incontestable [65]. Perception of the opportunity structure remains pivotal and, until that opportunity window opens more widely through better reward for technical qualification, it is difficult to see how any significant change will occur. Middle-income status may be achieved by 2030 but there is still likely to be large sectors of the population, marginalized in poverty with obvious consequences for their wellbeing [66].

11. Conclusion

Within this setting of overall growth in the economy and in school enrollments no longer principally at primary and basic school levels but at secondary and higher levels, by 2017 the primary school enrollment reached 3, 300,000 [67]. The country had almost achieved its target of universal primary schooling. It was noted that this goal, though in sight, was still not achieved as the net enrollment rate of the age-relevant children was 80 percent and completion rate 79 percent [68]. Part of the reason entails high repetition and drop-out rates, low quality linked to poor infrastructure including high numbers of students in classrooms, insufficient numbers of teachers, lack of textbooks and free schooling in theory rather than in reality [69]. One could argue that the whole Zambian population has been included in gaining some degree of literacy at the primary level, leaving overall literacy at approximately 75 percent. This of course assumes that completion of primary or even basic school can be correlated with a satisfactory level of literacy [70].

While this emerges as an unquestionable achievement and the result of a long-time ambition, it has a major shadow. It does not provide the majority with the prospect of formal employment and the rewards associated with that. Instead, it leaves the country, like many other African countries, with 60 percent of the population of approximately 16 million marginalized. They are said to be in poverty of varying degrees, high level or extreme for 5 million and moderate for almost 8 million [71]. One might say that the education system that was originally thought to promote a prosperous nation with wealth equitably shared has delivered something very different.

Among other things, this means that, while 88 percent of students in primary school aspire to university education, only 3-4 percent have access to it. Though one might claim that the system offers equality of opportunity through its meritocratic system, is this true? The boy/girl from Matero who we mentioned at the outset has a much weaker chance of climbing the educational ladder not necessarily because he/she is less gifted but because he/she is located where he/she does not have the resources to enter the school system well equipped. He/she is unlikely to have had pre-school, educated parents, facility in speaking and reading English at home, which most of his/her well-to-do age-mates from more affluence parts of the city have and so they are likely to gain higher grades in the Grade VII test. This enables them to be admitted to the Catholic school which, like most Catholic schools, prides itself on good performance in meritocratic pro-privileged national league Tables [72]. The Matero boy/girl has to travel to where his/her schooling is likely to be less well resourced.

This trend is seen more widely where 37 percent of Grade I students reach Grade 9 or secondary school. Even if he/she finds him/herself in the 26 percent who reach Grade XII, College entry ranges at roughly 3 percent and there is almost no chance of having access to university [73]. Given this pattern that clearly favours the 'haves', we find that 77 percent of university students coming from the richest 10 percent of the population and they were assisted with state bursaries at tax-payers' cost [74].

As the overall rate of inclusion of the population at the primary level is to be commended so too is the overall expansion of those completing secondary and higher education in large part because of widespread development of private contributions so that the country now has five public and upward of 32 private universities and multiple colleges in concord with the human capital approach to the goal of middle-income status in 2030 [75]. However, without large-scale economic development and dramatic increase in the formal employment rate, what is likely to result, will be somewhat like we find in 2017 when the country had 85,000 or so teachers emerging from colleges, there was employment for 2,000 or so, leaving the country with ever larger numbers of marginalized college and university graduates [76]. The linear system, even modified by *Framework 2012,* still needs urgent and radical reform if it is to deliver not purely middle-income status for a fortunate few.

Despite the hopes of those who led the country after 1964 of creating a prosperous nation where the division between those who 'have' and those 'left out' or marginalized would be small, the modernization mode of schooling by which they strove to achieve this delivered a different outcome, dispelling the persistent myth of achieving equality through a meritocratic system. This was glimpsed early in the history of schooling in the country but adopting an alternative paradigm proved to be difficult not only for the state but even for faith-based public schools because of the power of a newly formed elite.

This discussion has recounted how the Zambian school system has marginalized a major part of the population from access to the kind of lifestyle that each person has reason to value. Government initially attempted to counteract this progressive exclusion of the majority through reform in the 1970s. It failed and resorted to a piece-meal solution along the lines of basic education for all. In the early part of the 21st century, after debt relief and a more buoyant economy, government invested in setting the school system on better footing. Though welcome, this has not confronted the social structure and the school system as part of it, marginalising the majority and frustrating its desire for an acceptably equitable level of well-being for every Zambian.

Author details

Brendan P. Carmody[1,2]

1 Institute of Education, University College, London

2 St. Mary's University, London

*Address all correspondence to: carmody.brendan4@gmail.com

References

[1] T. Gilead, "Education and the Logic of Economic Progress," *Journal of the Philosophy of Education* 46,1 (2012):113-131; P. B. Walters, "*Educational Change and National Economic Development*," *Harvard Educational Review* 51, 1 (1981): 94-106.

[2] K.D. Kaunda, *Humanism in Zambia and a Guide to Its Implementation* Part II (Lusaka: Government Printer, n.d.), 109-110.

[3] The education system was made up of primary Grades 1-7, secondary Form I-5 for many years, then in 1986, it changed to primary Grades 1-7, Basic Grades 1-9, high school, Grades 10-12; this was abandoned in 2011 and the system reverted to primary Grades 1-7.

[4] N. Noddings, *Happiness and Education* (Cambridge: Cambridge University Press, 2003), 74-93; A. Courtois, *Elite Schooling and Social Inequality: Privilege and Power in Ireland's Top Private Schools* (London: Palgrave Macmillan, 2018), 43,98.

[5] B. Carmody, "Secular and Sacred at Chikuni: 1905-1940," *Journal of Religion in Africa* XXI, 2 (1991): 140-142.

[6] B. Carmody, *Conversion and Jesuit Schooling in Zambia* (Leiden: E.J. Brill, 1992), 5-6.

[7] R. Clignet & P. Foster, *The Fortunate Few: A study of secondary schools in the Ivory Coast* (Evanston IL: North Western University Press, 1966).

[8] J. Gremillion, *The Gospel of Peace and Justice* (New York: Orbis, 1992).

[9] .P. Riordan, *A Grammar of the Common Good* (London: Continuum, 2008).

[10] Pope Paul VI, *Populorum Progresssio* (New York: Paulist Press, 1967); D. Torevell, "Liberation, Catholic Education and the Nature of Theology: an essay to assist Catholic teachers with problems in this field," *International Studies in Catholic Education* 5,2 (2013): 318-332.

[11] C.J. Beirne, "Jesuit education for justice: the Collegio in El Salvador, 1968-1984," *Harvard Educational Review* 55 (1985): 1-19.

[12] *Deus Caritas Est: Encyclical Letter of Benedict XVI* (London: CTS, 2006):28.

[13] *The Catholic School* (Washington D.C.: Catholic Confernce, n.d.), Para 58.

[14] Q. Woden, "How well do Catholic and other Faith-Based Schools Serve the Poor? A Study with special reference to Africa: part I: Schooling," *International Studies in Catholic Education* 11, 1 (2019):4-23.

[15] E. H. Berman, *African Reactions to Mission Education* (New York: Teachers College Press, 1975), xi.

[16] N. P. Stromquist, "Education: A Journey Toward Equality and Equity," *Harvard Educational Review* 75,1 (2005): 93-97.

[17] M. J. Kelly, *Education in a Declining Economy: The Case of Zambia* (Washington D.C: The World Bank, 1991), 13.

[18] *Educating Our Future* (Lusaka: Ministry of Education, 1996), 9.

[19] K. Kaunda, *Humanism* Part II, 6.

[20] Gilead, "Education and the Logic of Economic Progress," 113-131.

[21] W.W. Rostow, *Stages of Economic Growth* (London: Cambridge University Press, 1962).

[22] T. W. Shultz, *Investing in People* (Berkeley: University of California Press, 1981)

[23] B. Carmody, *The Evolution of Education in Zambia* (Lusaka: Bookworld Publications, 2004): 27-29.

[24] Carmody, *The Evolution of Education in Zambia,* 29.

[25] T. Scudder & E. Colson, *Secondary Education and the formation of an elite: the impact of education in Gwembe district, Zambia* (New York: Academic Press, 1980).

[26] A. G. Frank, "The development of underdevelopment," in J.D. Cockcroft (Ed.), *Dependence and Development: Latin America's Political Economy* (New York: Anchor, 1972); Stromquist, "Education: A Journey Toward Equality and Equity," 93.

[27] Carmody, *The Evolution of Education in Zambia*, 33-35; B. Carmody, "Denominational Secondary Schooling in Post-Independent Zambia: A Case Study," *African Affairs* 89, 355 (1990): 253.

[28] *Education for Development: Draft Statement on Educational Reform* (Lusaka: Ministry of Education, 1976).

[29] *Education for Development,*1.

[30] P. H. Coombs, *The World Crisis in Education: The View from the Eighties* (New York: Oxford University Press, 1985), 213; K. Blakemore & B. Cooksey, *A Sociology of Education for Africa* (London: George Allen & Unwin, 1982), 90-93.

[31] *Educational Reform: Proposals and Recommendations* (Lusaka: Ministry of Education, 1977).

[32] Blakemore & Cooksey, *A Sociology of Education for Africa*, 83; Coombs, *The World Crisis in Education*, 218; G.F. Lungu, "Instrumentalism and educational policy-making in post-Independent Zambia," *Comparative Education* 21,3 (1985): 292; P. Bourdieu and J. Passeron, *Reproduction in eduction, society and culture* (London: Sage, 1977).

[33] Scudder & Colson, *Secondary Education and the formation of an elite: the impact of education in Gwembe district, Zambia*.

[34] M. Larmer, M. Hinfelaar, B.J. Phiri, L. Schumacher & M. Szeftel, "Introduction," *Journal of Southern African Studies* 40,5 (2014): 902-903; G.F. Lungu, "The Church, Labour and the Press in Zambia: the role of critical observers in a one-party state," *African Affairs* 83, 240 (1986): 385-410.

[35] M. Mwalimu, "Education and the Economy: Achievements and Shortfalls in Independent Zambia, 1964-2014," *Journal of Southern African Studies* 40, 5 (2014): 1100.

[36] Blakemore & Cooksey, *A Sociology of Education for Africa*, 19.

[37] *The Provision of Education for All(Lusaka: University of Zambia, 1986),* 181.

[38] G. Lungwangwa, "The Rationale for Basic Education in Developing Countries: a critique of the ideology in Education," *Critical Arts* 4 (1988):15.

[39] C. Harber (Ed.), *Education in Southern Africa* (London: Bloomsbury, 2013), 32,40,63.

[40] *The Provision of Education for All,* 290.

[41] Carmody, *The Evolution of education in Zambia*, 74.

[42] M. Mwalimu, "Education and the Economy: Achievements and Shortfalls

in Independent Zambia, 1964-2014," 1009.

[43] J. Ogbu, *The Next Generation* (New York: Academic Press, 1974).

[44] *Will the Poor Go to School* (Report by Oxfam-Zambia, 2001): 5-6.

[45] *Education in Zambia 2002: Situational Analysis* (Lusaka: Ministry of Education, 2002):21; M. Bajaj, "International Perspectives on Education and Employment in the Zambian Copperbelt," *Comparative Education Review* 54, 2 (2010): 181.

[46] M.J.Kelly and E. Banda-Sinkala, "Educational Disabilities of Vulnerable Children in Zambia," in M. J. Kelly, *The Origins and Development of Education* (Lusaka: Image Publications, 1999), 278-279.

[47] Mwalimu, "Education and the Economy..."1100.

[48] *Education Public Expenditure Review in Zambia* (Washington D.C: World Bank, 2015),10.

[49] Bajaj, "International Perspectives on Education and Employment in the Zambian Copperbelt," 181.

[50] *Education Public Expenditure Review,* 25.

[51] Bajaj, "International Perspectives on Education and Employment in the Zambian Copperbelt,"187; P.H. Coombs, *The World Crisis in Education: a view from the Eighties*, 10.

[52] Carmody, *The Evolution of Education in Zambia*, 142.

[53] B. Carmody, "The Catholic school and social justice in Africa: a Zambian case study," *Paedagogica Historica* 52,5 (2016): 562; Larmer et al, "Introduction," *Journal of Southern African Studies* 40,5 (2014): 933; Coombs, *The World Crisis in Education,* 135, 181.

[54] *Education Public Expenditure Review,* 31.

[55] Mwalimu, "Education and the Economy: Achievements and Shortfalls in Independent Zambia, 1102; Carmody, *The Evolution of education in Zambia*, 145.

[56] M.A.M. Thomas, C.M. Thomas, E.E. Lefebre, "Dissecting the teacher monolith: Experiences of beginning basic teachers in Zambia," *International Journal of Educational Development* 38 (2014): 39-46; Stromquist, "Education: A Journey Toward Equality and Equity," 101.

[57] Thomas et al., "Dissecting the teacher monolith...," 39.

[58] Carmody, *The Evolution of education in Zambia*, 66-67; Bajaj, "International Perspectives on Education and Employment in the Zambian Copperbelt,"181.

[59] *2008 Educational Statistical Bulletin* (Lusaka: Ministry of Education, 2008), 29.

[60] *2008 Educational Statistical Bulletin*, 15.

[61] *Education Public Expenditure Review,* 65-75; Mwalimu, "Education and the Economy: Achievements and Shortfalls in Independent Zambia, 1106.

[62] *Education Curriculum Framework 2012* (Lusaka: Ministry of Education, Science, Vocational Training and Early Education, 2012).

[63] Harber, *Education in Southern Africa*, 5.91,380; Stromquist, "Education: A Journey Toward Equality and Equity," 100.

[64] *Education Public Expenditure Review,*24-28, 91.

[65] *Education Public Expenditure Review,* 41.

[66] V. Seshemani, "Achieving middle-income status by 2030: Is this the most appropriate objective for Zambia?" *Zambia Social Science Journal* 1,2 (2010): 189-202.

[67] *Education Statistics Bulletin (2015)* (Lusaka: Ministry of Education, 2017), 21.

[68] *Education Public Expenditure Review in Zambia* (Washington D.C: World Bank, 2015), 2-3.

[69] *Education Public Expenditure Review, 3.*

[70] Harber, *Education in Southern Africa*, 11-12. B. Piper, "Editor's Review," *Harvard Educational Review* 77,1 (2007)103; Bajaj, "International Perspectives on Education and Employment in the Zambian Copperbelt,"193.

[71] *Education Public Expenditure Review,* 1; C. Wolhuter (Ed.), *Education in East and Central Africa* (London: Bloomsbury. 2014), 16, 71, 113.

[72] B. Carmody, "The Catholic School and Social Justice in Africa: a Zambian case study," *Paedagogica Historica* 52, 5 (2016): 559-574; Noddings, *Happiness and Education,* 74-93.

[73] *Education Public Expenditure Review,* 44, 91.

[74] *Education Public Expenditure Review,* 44; Mwalimu, "Education and the Economy: Achievements and Shortfalls in Independent Zambia, 1105.

[75] *Education Public Expenditure Review,* 23; Wolhuter, Education in East and Central Africa, 53,147;

[76] Zambian Eye (23 September 2017); Bajaj, "International Perspectives on Education and Employment in the Zambian Copperbelt,"187, 193.

Chapter 9

Living with Violence and Its Relationship with Executive Function in Childhood and Adolescence: Literature Review

Daniela Sacramento Zanini, Larissa de Oliveira e Ferreira and Karina Ferreira Leao Junqueira

Abstract

The purpose of this article is to conduct a literature review of studies that have investigated the relationship between violence and the development of executive function (EF) in children and adolescents. A search was carried out in the PsycINFO, PubMed/Medline, BVS, Lilacs, Web of Science, Scopus, and Gale databases with the following descriptors; violence, executive functions, child, children, adolescence, an adolescent. A total of 486 articles, published in the last 10 years, were found. After reading the abstracts and considering the inclusion and exclusion criteria, eight articles remain that are related to the topic. It was found that all the studies investigated the relationship of abuse in children and adolescents. Diversity was also observed in terms of the EF components evaluated as well as in the instruments for assessing EF. Moreover, seven of the eight studies established that victimization impairs EF.

Keywords: executive function, violence, children and adolescents

1. Introduction

Violence has become an issue of public health, responsible for deaths and illnesses, leaving in its wake consequences for all age groups in the population. Intentionality is one of the more complex elements in the concept of violence, however, the World Health Organization (WHO) explains that any act causing implications for an individual's health is considered a violent act, even when sustained by the culture or when there was an intention to use force without the intention to cause harm [1].

As far as the typology is concerned, violence is divided into three types: self-inflicted, interpersonal, and collective. Self-inflicted violence is subdivided into suicidal behavior and self-abuse; collective violence, into social, political, and economic; lastly, interpersonal, divided into two subcategories: violence within the family or by a close partner, which mostly occurs between family members, and community violence, which takes place among people who are unrelated [2].

With regard to the nature of violent acts, these may be classified as physical, sexual, psychological, deprivation or abandonment. The four types of violent act occur in each of the main categories and subcategories, except for self-inflicted violence. Violence towards children, committed inside the home, for example, may include physical, sexual, or psychological abuse, as well as negligence or abandonment [3].

Specifically, with regard to children and adolescents, violent acts (physical, sexual, psychological, negligent) are called maltreatment and refer to various forms of violence, in the majority of cases with events being repeated and committed by someone close or the guardian of the child or adolescent [4].

Studies into violence, conducted by Finkelhor et al. [5], assert that living with or experiencing situations of violence, with the particular potential to cause trauma, is called victimization. Studies into victimization describe five types of violence: victimization through conventional crime, victimization through maltreatment, victimization by peers, sexual victimization and indirect, witnessed victimization.

Victimization through conventional crime is commonly identified by the police authorities as, for example, assault, theft, vandalism, and prejudice. As for violence through maltreatment, this is detected through living with situations of violence directly related to the family or to guardians. This type of victimization also includes negligence, physical and psychological abuse, in the form of depriving children and/or adolescents of basic necessities like food and hygiene. Victimization by peers is characterized by the aggression that occurs by individuals within the same age group, normally among students. In this respect, aggression through the practice of bullying is also taken into account as well as attacks by groups and physical and psychological violence. Sexual victimization relates to aggression related to issues of sexuality. For Finkelhor et al. [5], sexual victimization is more than just penetration, it also includes lewd acts without the consent of the individual or even with consent where the children are not old enough to be responsible for their choices; this also encompasses sexual aggression by an adult, by peers, sexual harassment, rape or attempted rape and sexually-related verbal harassment. Lastly, indirect victimization refers to the witnessing of violence suffered by others, and this also covers issues such as witnessing domestic violence, seeing parents attack siblings or their spouses, witnessing attacks, robberies, homicides, shootings, terrorism, and exposure to ethnic conflict.

In epidemiological terms, studies show that approximately 40 million children in the world, under the age of 15, have suffered abuse and negligence [1] and, in the USA, between 25% and 66% of children and adolescents are exposed to traumatic events during childhood [6, 7]. As far as Brazil is concerned, a survey by the Brazilian Center for Latin American Studies, based on the Ministry of Health's Mortality Information System (SIM), shows that the number of homicides of teenagers, between 1980 and 2010, rose 346%.

Brazilian researcher that investigates violence directed against children and adolescents point to alarming data. According to the National Human Rights Ombudsman, 58.9% of the complaints received via channels such as Dial 100 refer to some type of violence against children and adolescents. The main types of violence reported are mistreatment: negligence (61,416), psychological violence (39,561), and physical violence (33,105). In 2017 alone, there were 84,049 reports of physical violence and, in the previous year, there were 76,171. In this sense, the data indicate that 68% of Brazilian children and adolescents aged up to 14 years, which is equivalent to 30.3 million children and adolescents, have already suffered corporal violence at home [8].

An exploratory/descriptive desk study conducted by Júnior et al. [9], analyzed the characterization of cases of domestic violence against children and adolescents in the Brazilian city of Volta Redonda, situated in the state of Rio de Janeiro. The investigation was carried out based on an analysis of the patient records of registered children and adolescents cared for as victims of maltreatment by parents, relatives, and/or guardians in the city's Specialized Social Welfare Reference Center (CREAS). The results indicated that, of the 210 patient records analyzed, 29% were victims of physical violence, 29% sexual violence, 29% were linked to negligence and 13% were cases of psychological violence. Although this study cannot be generalized as it makes use of a convenience sample, some important points were deliberated. The prevalence of the identification of physical violence, as it leaves marks on the body, and sexual violence, as it causes significant harm to the victims' health, is capable of mobilizing more the child protection institutions and society in general, which probably explains the higher volumes of identification. As for negligence, though difficult to identify, as it involves the economic and social aspects of each family or social group, detection is possible when there is already contact between the social institutions and the families in situations of risk and vulnerability. On the other hand, psychological violence, which accounted for the smallest percentage of identification, requires children's welfare professionals to redouble their attention because the indicators of its manifestation are not so straightforward, however, the consequences are equally serious for the victims' mental health.

One study conducted by Lin et al. [10] investigate the link between serious child abuse and cerebral activation based on Magnetic Resonance Imaging examinations during a sustained attentional task. A total of 70 individuals (13 to 20 years old) took part, divided into three groups: history of abuse before 12 years old; psychiatric control group (no maltreatment but with psychiatric disorders); control group (no maltreatment, no psychological disorders). The results indicated that the participants exposed to child abuse exhibited results that show that the longer the youngster suffered abuse, the worse the performance in capacity to maintain sustained attention.

Another important piece of data indicates that, according to the Ministry of Women, Family and Human Rights (MMFDH), of the accusations received via Helpline 100 in 2018, over 17,000 were related to sexual abuse and sexual exploitation involving children and adolescents. Thus, based on the data presented and seeking protective measures for children and adolescents, in Brazil, the Child and Adolescent Statute (ECA) is regarded as one of the most advanced pieces of legislation in the world in terms of child protection [11]. Among the general clauses, the law establishes full protection for children and adolescents, considering that children, for the purposes of the law, are those aged under 12 while adolescents are those aged between 12 and 18 years. In terms of protection against violence, article 5 of the ECA states that no child or adolescent shall be the object of any form of negligence, discrimination, exploitation, violence, cruelty, or oppression and that any attempt, through commission or omission, against their fundamental rights must be punished in accordance with the law. Despite the ECA and the penalties it imposes on people who commit violence against children and adolescents, the percentage of victims within this age group is still significant.

Despite the ECA being a statute that provides for severe infractions for those who are aggressors, the number of victimizations is still significant. The aim of the ECA, therefore, is the full protection of children and adolescents, seeking to guarantee their cognitive, psychosocial, and physical development. The dividing line between child and adolescent is important, mainly as it considers that significant, important differences exist during each period of their lives [12].

Development in childhood is characterized by constant processes of development in terms of cognitive function and social skills. In the third stage of childhood, between six and 11 years of age, cognitive development is seen as an increase in cognitive skills that permits an improvement in the ability to learn as well as preparation for academic performance. In terms of psychosocial development, relationships between peers, schoolmates, and others take on fundamental importance. In adolescence, interest in peer relationships remains strong, however, with a greater concern to belong to a group, which may exert positive or negative influences. Cognitive development is characterized by the ability to think in abstract terms, but immature thinking persists in some attitudes and conduct, with more impulsive behavior [12]. Situations of violence may adversely affect this important period of development, causing impairment of cognitive, social, emotional skills and, consequently, may compromise the quality of life of victimized subjects.

With regard to the damage to quality of life, for victimized children, a study by Matos, Pinto, and Stelko-Pereira [13], which aimed to investigate the existence of a possible connection between exposure to sexual abuse in childhood and inferior quality of life in university students, noted that childhood sexual abuse is negatively associated with quality of life in adults. The results of another study, conducted by Dias [14], although investigating a different age group, specifically relating to the impact of violence on the quality of life of adult females, showed that violence exerts a negative impact on the quality of life of victims and also generates physical trauma, posttraumatic stress disorder, stress, and depression.

Studies into the relationship of experience of violence in childhood and adolescence have increased as a result of the recognition of the dimensions of the phenomenon as a serious public health problem, on account of the high index and the consequences they have for the physical, psychological and cognitive health of people who suffer violence [15]. In order to identify victimization, for the most part, studies look to institutions that protect victimized children, as well as instruments (questionnaires and/or scales) that can be answered by the parents/guardians or by the child or adolescent him/herself. The instruments most frequently employed are the Child Maltreatment Questionnaire, Child Trauma Questionnaire, and Juvenile Victimization Questionnaire [4, 10, 16, 17]. The last two instruments in this list include validity studies in the national context conducted by Grassi-Oliveira et al. [18] and Faria and Zanini [19], respectively, and are not instruments restricted to the use of psychologists.

Despite the variety in the way victimization is identified, studies have shown impairment to cognitive functions in this age group [4, 10, 20]. However, there are still very few studies available that have sought to investigate the impact of violence specifically on executive functions.

Executive function (EF) refers to the processes called upon whenever it is necessary to focus attention, manage and control behavior or action towards a goal, evaluate the efficiency of this behavior, and readjust strategy when required. Thus it is possible to assert that the human capacity to adapt to different situations is heavily associated with good executive function [21–24].

In spite of the agreement between the theoretical models that EF is important for good brain function, insofar as it relates to its definition and component structure, there seems to be a divergence in ideas [14, 25–27]. Thus, several different EF models have been developed and studied.

One of the more influential theories about EF proposes the association between the frontal lobes, their principal connections, and the Supervisory Attentional System (SAS). SAS is a model developed by Norman and Shallice [28] and describes EF as a specific system in the processing of information, which takes place based on two processes. An automatic process is the ability to automatically select responses based on information in an existing repertoire. The controlled process is identified as the modification or even the construction of new responses, including decision-making, mental flexibility, inhibitory control, and planning [28, 29]. In this regard, there are some studies about the relationship of violence with EF [10, 30] which used attention as a component of EF.

One widely accepted model is that of Miyaki et al. [31], for whom EF is composed of three basic components or nuclear EFs, namely: working memory (WM), cognitive flexibility (CF), and inhibitory control (IC). Subsequently, Diamond [21] carried out a new study corroborating the idea that three nuclear EFs exist, but that they are the basis for the development of more complex components such as planning, deductive reasoning, and problem resolution, subsequently designated complex executive functions. For a better understanding of the model, it is necessary to define each of these components.

IC involves the ability to control the behaviors of attention, thoughts, and emotions, inhibiting an automatic behavior or a distraction and, instead of generating said behavior, do what is most appropriate or necessary [22]. WM is defined as the ability to keep information in one's mind and deal with it over a short period of time, enabling understanding, learning, and reasoning, as well as problem resolution [32]. CF involves the capacity to change perspectives, alternate attentional focus, favoring the ability to adapt to the environment, enabling the individual to evaluate his/her performance in a particular situation, seeking to comply with rules, and problem resolution [22, 33]. With regard to complex EFs, planning involves the ability, based around an initial starting point, to set an objective, define the best ways to achieve it, organize the necessary steps to this end, analyze the efficacy and, if necessary, adjust the execution [22]. Problem resolution involves the ability to create and test solutions for conflicts, through mental representation, in the planning and implementation of strategies and monitoring [34].

Another skill developed from the three nuclear components is decision-making, crucial for day-to-day functioning because it involves a process of choice of one among many alternatives in situations that include uncertainty, generally guided by an emotional or motivational component. During decision-making, other EF components are involved like operational memory, cognitive flexibility, inhibitory control, and planning [23, 34].

Regarding the development of EF in the early years of life, it is considered a unitary construct, that is to say, in this phase it is not possible to distinguish between each component, however, it is already possible to identify an improvement in the performance of the components in the first year of life [35].

From school age, the development of operational memory and cognitive flexibility is relatively linear; in this period, the EF components appear in sequence: firstly working memory, then inhibitory control. The two components in combination permit the development of cognitive flexibility [23, 36].

Adolescence is characterized by an increase in impulsiveness and, consequently, by a pattern of immediatist choices, changes in the course of action without making a conscience judgment, unintended behaviors, and a tendency to act without planning. All these aspects lead to risk-taking behavior without evaluating the consequences, suggesting a lesser capacity for self-regulation and inhibitory control [23].

WM is an essential ability in learning, both in childhood and in adolescence and, although there are a series of abilities required for learning, there is evidence that working memory is one of the best predictors of performance at school [37, 38]. In this regard, it is important to stress that the development of EF is directly related to the ability of children and adolescents in the learning processes, as well as the ability to adapt to new situations.

As EF is important for the learning processes, the evaluation of this function must investigate, in minute detail, if each of the components is developing as expected. There are specific batteries for its evaluation, such as the Behavioral Assessment of the Dysexecutive Syndrome (BADS) and the Delis Kaplan Executive Function System (D-KEFS). These batteries perform an overall evaluation of EF and serve a population ranging in age from eight to 87 years.

There are several favorable psychological tests, which evaluate EF, as well as instruments validated for use. The Wisconsin Card Test, for example, is used to evaluate EF, specifically cognitive flexibility, as well as Trail Making Test and the Five Digit Test (FDT). To evaluate WM, the WISC-IV subtests are used, such as digit span and numbers and letters sequencing and, to evaluate inhibitory control, FDT, Stroop Test, and the Hayling Test are used. On the one hand, the wide variety of tests to evaluate EF permits a full investigation based on the collection of data from all the components, however, with regard to the comparison of data in studies, it may make analysis difficult as the studies use different instruments and tests.

Despite the diversity, in the way, the data is collected, either for identifying violence or evaluating EF, international studies point out the consequences of victimization for children and adolescents. Some studies have investigated the consequences of short- and long-term violence with victims who presented with a condition indicative of posttraumatic stress disorder, psychiatric disorders, or the use of illicit substances such as alcohol and drugs [39–43]. Other studies have shown that victimization as a result of maltreatment, as well as sexual victimization, may impair the development of EF in terms of the components of working memory, cognitive flexibility, and inhibitory control [39, 41, 44, 45].

So, based on the data presented, the present study aimed to perform a literature review of the literature concerning studies that investigated the relationship between living with violence and the development of EF in children and adolescents, over the last 10 years. It also intends to demonstrate how these impairments can affect the quality of life of these children and adolescents.

2. Method

2.1 Materials

Articles in scientific reviews, published within the last 10 years, which sought to assess the relationship between living with violence and executive function in children and adolescents aged between six and 16, located in the following databases: PsycINFO, Pubmed/Medline, BVS, Lilacs, Web of Science, Scopus and Gale.

2.2 Procedures

In order to carry out this literature review, the following databases were used: PsycINFO, Pubmed/Medline, BVS, Lilacs, Web of Science, Scopus, and Gale, with articles, published up to October 2019. In these databases, the potentially relevant documents were selected using the following descriptors: executive functions, violence, child, children, adolescent, and adolescence, inserting the *and.* Boolean operator between the descriptors:

Studies between 2009 and October 2019 were accepted, reviewed by peers, and published in the English, Spanish and Portuguese languages. Initially, 486 articles were located, of which 200 were repeated articles. After a reading of the titles and abstracts of the remaining 286 articles, 221 were excluded, in accordance with the following criteria: articles that were not available in their entirety (16), that had no connection with the proposed topic (172), comprising longitudinal studies (7), with a target demographic of subjects over 16 years of age (10), with a target demographic of subjects under 6 years of age (11), related to the use of illicit drugs (5). A total of 65 articles remained, selected for a full-text reading, to be subsequently included or excluded in accordance with the following criteria:

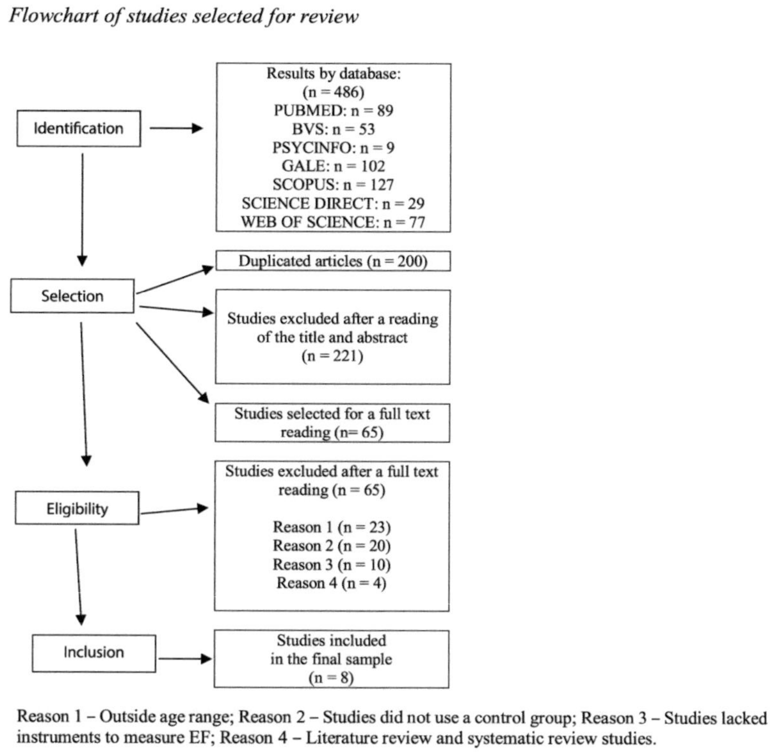

Figure 1.
Flowchart of studies selected for review.

Inclusion criteria: (1) articles that investigated the relationship between violence and EF, (2) articles with a target demographic between six and 16 years of age, (3) studies with a control group. Exclusion criteria: duplicated articles (2), articles not available in full, (3) articles with a target demographic under 6 years of age, (4) articles that did not indicate the instruments used to evaluate EF. Based on the final analysis of the selection, the studies were characterized by author and year of publication, objective, age range of target demographic, type/nature of violence, instruments used, evaluated EF components and results. **Figure 1** represents the detailed flowchart of the study selection process.

Figure 1 indicates that the initial search of the databases identified 486 files. After applying inclusion and exclusion criteria, 65 articles remained for full-text reading. After the reading, the following studies were excluded: outside the studied age range (n = 25), those that did not have a control group (n = 23), those without instruments to measure EF (n = 13), and those which were literature or systematic reviews (n = 4), leaving a total of eight articles.

3. Results

There follow a series of tables with the results obtained in this review study. **Table 1** describes the eight articles selected according to the inclusion criteria, identifying the authors, number of participants, age group, and study objectives.

The results displayed in **Table 1** show that the number of participants ranged from 26 to 1851. As far as the age range is concerned, just one study analyzed only children [30], three investigated both children and adolescents [39, 45, 46] and four studies investigated adolescents [10, 16, 17, 47]. With regard to the objectives

Authors	Participants	Objective
De Bellis et al. [30]	Children (7 and 8 years old)	To investigate impairment in cognitive functions in neglected and sexually abused children. The children were divided into three groups: neglected and with symptoms of PTSD; neglected but no PTSD, children neither neglected nor PTSD (control group). The following cognitive domains were investigated: IQ, reading, math, fine-motor coordination, speech, visuospatial perception, memory, attention/ executive function.
Nooner et al. [45]	202 children (11 and 12 years old).	To investigate the impact of maltreatment on cognitive functions, comparing boy and girl victims. The cognitive functions investigated were: attention, speech, memory, intelligence, EF, and academic performance (reading, writing). The children were divided into 4 groups: boys with and without maltreatment; girls with and without maltreatment.
Spann et al. [16]	30 adolescents (12 to 17 years old).	To investigate the relationship between maltreatment and EF, specifically cognitive flexibility in adolescents without psychiatric disorders. The adolescents, divided into two groups: with and without a history of maltreatment.
Borges and Dell'Aglio [39]	26 children and adolescents (8 to 13 years old)	To identify the manifestation of symptoms of PTSD and impairment of attention, verbal memory, cognitive flexibility/ executive function in girls that suffered sexual abuse. Divided into 2 groups: girls who were victims of sexual abuse and girls without a history of sexual abuse.
Smith et al. [46]	80 adolescents (11 to 18 years old)	To investigate if adolescents who suffered maltreatment exhibited worse performance in EF than the group which did not suffer maltreatment. Divided into 2 groups; with and without maltreatment.
Tran et al. [17]	1851 children and adolescents (12 to 17 years old)	Cross-sectional study investigating associations between different forms of maltreatment and emotional function, cognitive function, physical health, as well as the effects of the moderation of ethnicity and gender. Divided into 2 groups, with and without maltreatment.
Lim et al. [10]	70 adolescents (13 to 20 years old)	To investigate the link between serious child abuse and cerebral activation based on Magnetic Resonance Imaging examinations during a sustained attentional task. History of abuse before 12 years old; psychiatric control group (no maltreatment but with psychiatric disorders); control group (no maltreatment, no psychological disorders).
Vasilevski and Tucker [47]	82 children and adolescents (12 to 16 years of age)	To investigate to what extent maltreatment impacts cognitive performance, including the EF of adolescents who suffered maltreatment. Divided into two groups: the first composed of adolescents who suffered severe maltreatment and the second, adolescents who did not suffer any maltreatment.

Table 1.
Authors, Participants, and Objective of the study.

of the studies, it was possible to observe that all the articles included studies related to maltreatment. Two studies sought to identify a correlation between maltreatment, cognitive/executive functions, and Post Traumatic Stress Syndrome (PTSD) [30, 39], and one sought to identify the difference in the impact of maltreatment in adolescents with psychiatric disorders [10].

Table 2 shows that the most studied form of violence is interpersonal based on an investigation into maltreatment, however, several articles investigated specific types of maltreatment, namely negligence, physical abuse, sexual abuse, emotional

Authors	Type of violence	Investigation instrument
De Bellis et al. [30]	Negligence (excludes sexual abuse).	*Department of Social Services (DSS).*
Nooner et al. [45]	Maltreatment, negligence, physical abuse, sexual abuse, witnessing interpersonal violence at home, and emotional abuse.	*Child Protection Service (agency).*
Borges and Dell'Aglio [39]	Sexual abuse	Reference services for sexually abused children.
Spann et al. [16]	Physical abuse, emotional abuse, and negligence.	*Childhood Trauma Questionnaire* (CTQ).
Smith et al. [46]	Physical, sexual, or emotional abuse, negligence, and domestic violence.	Collection of records from teachers and tutors.
Lim et al. [10]	Severe child abuse.	*Childhood Trauma Questionnaire* (CTQ).
Tran et al. [17]	Physical abuse, sexual abuse, and negligence.	*Child Maltreatment Questionnaire*
Vasilevski and Tucker [47]	Maltreatment	*State government of Victoria, Department of human services*

Table 2.
Authors, types of violence, and instruments employed.

abuse, and witnessed violence. Five articles investigated negligence ([30]; Nooner et al. [45]; [16, 17, 46]); four studies investigated physical abuse [16, 17, 45, 46]; four, sexual abuse [17, 39, 45, 46]; two, emotional abuse [45, 46]; two, domestic violence [45, 46]; and one article investigated maltreatment, without specifying the nature thereof [47].

As for the way to identify violence, five studies recruited children or adolescents from institutions or agencies responsible for caring for victimized children and/or adolescents [30, 39, 45–47], two studies used the Child Trauma Questionnaire [10, 16] and one the Child Maltreatment Questionnaire [17]. Both instruments are self-report inventories composed of items to identify emotional, physical, or sexual abuse, and negligence in children and adolescents.

The results observed in **Table 3** show that the components of EF evaluated in six of the eight studies agree to the Miyake et al. [31] model that considers cognitive flexibility, working memory, and inhibitory control as the basic components for the evaluation of EF, but only one study evaluated the three components in conjunction [46]. Two studies evaluated two components: working memory and cognitive flexibility [39, 47]; a further two studies only analyzed cognitive flexibility [16, 45]; and one study only evaluated WM [17]. Two studies [10, 30] considered the EF model of Norman and Shallice [28], who describe EF as a unique system of cognitive functions, named the Supervisory Attentional System (SAS).

As far as the EF measurement instruments are concerned, it was possible to identify diversity. For the evaluation of CF, the following tests were employed: *Wisconsin Test Card*, *Trail Making Part B,* and the WISC III and WISC IV digit span backward and number and letter sequences subtests [16, 45, 47]; for the evaluation of WM, the following tests were performed: *Listening Recall Task* and the *Odd-One-Out Task*, *Digit Span Task*, WISC IV subtests (digit span forward and number and letter sequences), *Trail Making Part A* [17, 39, 46]. To analyze IC, the Verbal Inhibition/Motor Inhibition task from the D-KEFS Color-Word Interference Test was used [46].

Authors	Instruments, respective EF components	Results
De Bellis et al. [30]	*Conners' Continuous Performance Test-II.* Sustained attention.	Neglected children demonstrated a significantly worse performance in sustained attention, memory, planning and problem resolution.
Nooner et al. [45]	*Wisconsin Card Sorting Test.* Cognitive flexibility.	Boys who suffered maltreatment demonstrated worse EF performance than girls who suffered maltreatment and boys in the control group.
Borges & Dell'Aglio [39]	WISC-III digit span forward and backward; *Trail Making Test Part A and B.* Working memory and cognitive flexibility.	No differences were found between the groups in terms of working memory and cognitive flexibility.
Spann et al. [16]	*Wisconsin Card Test.* Cognitive flexibility.	Adolescents who suffered physical abuse and negligence showed worse performance in cognitive performance.
Smith et al. [46]	*Listening Recall Task* and the *Odd-One-Out Task; (Delis–Kaplan Executive Function), Verbal Inhibition/Motor Inhibition task (D-KEFS Color-Word Interference Test).* Working memory, inhibitory control, and cognitive flexibility.	Adolescents who suffered maltreatment demonstrated worse performance in working memory, fluency, and inhibition, however, cognitive flexibility was not affected in comparison with the control group.
Lim et al. [10]	*Sustained Attention Task.* Sustained attention.	Participants exposed to child abuse exhibited results that show that the longer the youngster suffered abuse, the worse the performance in capacity to maintain sustained attention.
Tran et al. [17]	*Digit Span Task.* Operational memory.	The experience of sexual abuse and negligence throughout their lives were related to worse performance with operational memory.
Vasilevski and Tucker [47]	WISC-IV. Working memory, cognitive flexibility, and executive function.	The results showed that the group of adolescents that suffered maltreatment demonstrated impaired EF, attention, and working memory.

Table 3.
Authors, Instruments, and Results.

As for the results of the articles, only one of the studies was unable to find significant correlations between maltreatment, specifically, sexual abuse and EF [39]. The remaining seven studies [16, 17, 45–47] noted impairment with EF based on the components evaluated, namely: WM, CF, and IC, as well as in attention [10, 30], in children and adolescents suffering maltreatment.

4. Discussion

The present study, the aim of which is to carry out a literature review of the literature in respect of the impact of violence on the executive functions of children and adolescents, outlines the picture of the last 10 years' studies on the topic, in both the domestic and international arenas.

The first issue to mention is that all the studies located investigated victimization through maltreatment; some of them specified the types (negligence, physical abuse, sexual abuse, emotional abuse, and the witnessing of interpersonal violence at home), while others considered maltreatment in a general sense. The prevalence of studies on the topic may be connected with the fact that epidemiological data indicate growing victimization through maltreatment in childhood and adolescence, as noted in Ending Violence in Childhood: Global Report [48]. Another aspect that should be considered is the typical development of the components of EF in this period between childhood and adolescence, extremely important for the processes of learning [36–38]. Thus, it has become important to investigate the situations which could interfere with this process, as is the case of violence.

The fact that there are four types of maltreatment might also explain the number of studies on this topic, as the specific studies consider sexual abuse and even physical abuse as maltreatment, including them in a single group. On the other hand, for Finkelhor et al. [5], sexual victimization is a form to be evaluated separately because sexual abuse includes lewd acts without the consent of the individual or even with the consent of children at an age when they cannot be responsible for their choices, including sexual aggression by an adult, by peers and sexually related verbal harassment. So, considering the study of victimization from Finkelhor et al. [5], sexual abuse would be in distinct study groups.

In this study, no articles were found concerning the impact of victimization through conventional crimes, violence by peers, and indirect or witnessed violence, which points to the scarcity of studies that evaluate other forms of victimization. In relation to indirect or witnessed violence, one study evaluates the impact of witnessing interpersonal violence, however, it does not include the witnessing of other forms of violence such as robberies, street attacks, and aggression between colleagues. In this sense, the results of the study conducted by Brancalhone et al. [49] indicate impairment of EF in the group of children victimized by bullying and also in those who witness it. They also pointed out that the impact of indirect violence or violence witnessed by children is evident in the course of their development, causing symptoms of depression and a drop in school performance.

As far as the evaluation of EF is concerned, only two studies [10, 30] used the model of Norman and Shallice [28], who describe EF as the Supervisory Attentional System (SAS) and, based on this, they considered sustained attention as a component of EF. The others used the model proposed by Miyake et al. [31], corroborating the literature that regards this as the model most used in both empirical and theoretical studies into EF. Just one study considered all three components, while the others used one or two components, considered responsible for the evaluation of EF. The result corroborates the literature, which is quite diverse in terms of the structure of the components [14, 26, 27], which results in complexity with the process of evaluating EF.

Despite the theoretical diversity, studies have shown that, for the most part, components of EF were impaired in children and adolescents who suffered maltreatment and only two of them presented different results. In the study by Borges & Dell'Aglio [39], girls aged between eight and 13 who suffered sexual abuse had no impairment of working memory and, in Smith et al. [46], adolescents who suffered maltreatment showed no CF impairment, but no studies were found with results that corroborate these data.

Working memory was the most studied component, appearing in four of the eight articles studied; of these four, three identified impairment with WM in children and adolescents victimized through maltreatment. Working memory is an ability essential to learning [37, 38, 50], so, the interest in investigating the impact of violence in this EF component can be justified. Studies have shown that maltreatment can impair WM in both childhood and adolescence and, consequently, the processes of learning, as well as academic performance.

As regards the instruments for EF evaluation, these are diverse, which could influence the comparison of the results found. To evaluate WM, the subtests *Listening Recall Task* and the *Odd-One-Out Task*, *Digit Span Task* were used in addition to the WISC IV tests (digit span forward and number and letter sequences) and Trail Making Part A. The WISC-IV Digit Span Forward and Number and Letter Sequences subtests are standardized and can be quickly applied. The Digit Span and the Trail Making Test A are standardized neuropsychological instruments, however, they are not regarded as psychological tests and, therefore, they are not used exclusively in psychology.

For the evaluation of CF, the following tests were used: *Wisconsin Test Card*, *Trail Making Part B* and the WISC III and WISC IV subtests Digit Span Backward and Number and Letter Sequences, all of which are quick to apply. To evaluate IC, the subtest Verbal Inhibition/Motor Inhibition task, from the D-KEFS Color-Word Interference Test, was used. The diversity of instruments used corroborates the literature, which points to the complex nature of evaluating EF and its components.

Studies show that children and adolescents are part of a vulnerable age group and, as a result, they are more subject to experiencing violence in its various forms. Self-report instruments that seek to identify the different types of violence, that is to say, those to which the children or adolescents themselves respond, are capable of analyzing the perception of living with violence in a more sensitive way or one that better approximates the extent to which this child or adolescent could be affected, and are thus considered to be more effective instruments, as they identify the perception of living with violence. In this regard, adolescents, the group with the largest number of studies, have greater capacity to identify this experience as their cognitive and emotional repertoire is better developed in terms of perception.

From childhood to adolescence, living with violence impairs the nuclear components of EF, namely working memory, cognitive flexibility, and inhibitory control, which are the basis for the development of the following complex components: planning, problem resolution, and decision-making. These components may be impaired, not to mention the processes of learning, of adaptation to situations in both cognitive and social aspects, which are characteristic of this age group, leading to difficulties that will be omnipresent in diverse situations throughout their lives.

Apart from the impairment of executive functions that the processes of victimization may cause in children and adolescents, these impairments may adversely affect the quality of life in this important age group. In this sense, a study conducted by the Center on the Developing Child, at Harvard [51], indicated that typical development in executive function skills help children to remember and follow instructions with various stages, to avoid distractions, control precipitous responses, adjust when the rules change, persist with the solution of problems and control long-term obligations which are directly associated with quality of life. Moreover, Matos et al. [13] noted that child sex abuse is negatively associated with quality of life in adulthood.

In short, the study notes the scarcity, mainly in the domestic setting, of studies investigating the relationship between living with violence and the development of EF. However, the studies that were found point out, for the most part, the impairments that living with violence may bring to the development of EF and with the processes of learning. It has become important than that future studies investigate not only experience of maltreatment but also that of other types of violence, justifying on scientific basis the need for investment in public policies that can avert living with violence, as well as in intervention policies and care for children and adolescents who are victims of violence.

Author details

Daniela Sacramento Zanini[1*], Larissa de Oliveira e Ferreira[2] and Karina Ferreira Leao Junqueira[3]

1 Center for Human Sciences, Department of Psychology, Pontifícia Catholic University of Goias, Goiania, Brazil

2 Department of Psychology, Estácio de Sá College of Goiás, Pontifícia Catholic University of Goias, Goiania, Brazil

3 Pontifícia Catholic University of Goias, Goiania, Brazil

*Address all correspondence to: dazanini@yahoo.com

References

[1] Krug EG, Mercy J, Dahlberg L, Mercy JA, Zwi AB, Lozano R. The World Report on Violence and Health. Geneva: World Health Organization; 2002

[2] OMS – Organización Mundial de la Salud. Informe mundial sobre la violencia y la salud: resumen. Oficina Regional para las Américas de la Organización Mundial de la Salud: Organización Panamericana de la Salud; 2002

[3] Dahlberg LL, Krug EG. Violência: um problema global de saúde pública. Ciência & Saúde Coletiva. 2007;**11**:1163-1178

[4] Silva RWS. Adaptação transcultural do *Juvenile Victimization Questionnaire R2* em amostra brasileira e mensuração de cortisol em crianças vítimas de maus-tratos [Dissertação de Mestrado não publicada]. Porto Alegre: Pontifícia Universidade Católica do Rio Grande do Sul; 2017

[5] Finkelhor D, Ormrod RK, Turner HA. Re-victimization patterns in a national longitudinal sample of children and youth. Child Abuse & Neglect. 2007;**31**:479-502

[6] Copeland WE, Keeler G, Angold A, Costello EJ. Traumatic events and posttraumatic stress in childhood. Archives of General Psychiatry. 2007;**64**(5):577-584. DOI: 10.1001/archpsyc.64.5.577

[7] Costello EJ, Erkanli A, Fairbank JA, Angold A. The prevalence of potentially traumatic events in childhood and adolescence. Journal Trauma Stress. 2002;**15**(2):99-112. DOI: 10.1023/A:1014851823163

[8] Brasil. Ministério da Sáude. Atlas da violência 2019. Brasília: Instituto de Pesquisa Econômica Aplicada, Fórum Brasileiro de Segurança Pública; 2019

[9] Júnior AAP, Borges VC, Santos JG. Caracterização da violência doméstica contra crianças e adolescentes e as estratégias interventivas em um município do Estado do Rio de Janeiro, Brasil. Caderno Saúde Coletiva. 2015;**23**(2):124-131. DOI: 10.1590/1414-462X201500020062

[10] Lim L, Hart H, Mehta MA, Simmons A, Mirza K, Rubia K. Neurofunctional abnormalities during sustained attention in severe childhood abuse. PLoS One. 2016;**11**(11):e0165547. DOI: 10.1371/journal.pone.0165547

[11] Silva LMP. Violência doméstica contra crianças e adolescentes. Associação Brasileira das Editoras Universitárias. 2002;**1**:1-238

[12] Papalaia DE, Feldman RD. O estudo do desenvolvimento humano. In: Papalaia EDE, Feldman RD, editors. Desenvolvimento humano. Porto Alegre: Artmed; 2013

[13] Matos KJN, Pinto FJM, Stelko-Pereira AC. Violência sexual na infância associa-se a qualidade de vida inferior em universitários [The sexual violence occurred in childhood is associated with undergraduate student's life quality]. Jornal Brasileiro de Psiquiatria. 2018;**67**(1):10-17. DOI: 10.1590/0047-2085000000178

[14] Dias NM, Gomes CMA, Reppold CT, Fioravanti-Bastos AC, Pires EU, Carreiro LRR, et al. Investigação da estrutura e composição das funções executivas: Análise de modelos teóricos. Revista Psicologia - Teoria e Prática. 2015;**17**(2):140-152. DOI: 10.15348/1980-6906/psicologia.v17n2p140-152

[15] Schraiber LBD, Oliveira AFLP, Couto MT. Violência e saúde: estudos científicos recentes. Revista Saúde Pública. 2006;**4**:112-125

[16] Spann MN, Mayes LC, Kalmar JH, Guiney J, Womer FY, Pittman B, et al. Childhood abuse and neglect and cognitive flexibility in adolescents. Child Neuropsychology. 2012;**18**(2): 182-189. DOI: 10.1080/09297049.2011.595400

[17] Tran NK, Marinus SRVB, Ijzendoorn HV, Alink LRA. The association between child maltreatment and emotional, cognitive, and physical health functioning in Vietnam. BMC Public Health. 2017;**17**:332. DOI: 10.1186/s12889-017-4258-z

[18] Grassi-Oliveira R, Stein LM, Pezzi JC. Tradução e validação de conteúdo da versão em português do Childhood Trauma Questionnaire. Revista de Saúde Pública. 2006;**40**(2):249-255. DOI: 10.1590/S0034-89102006000200010

[19] Faria MRGV, Zanini DS. Análise da compreensão dos itens do Questionário de Victimization (JVQ) após tradução para o português. In: Trabalho apresentado como Pôster na 63ª Reunião Anual da SBPC, 10 a 15 de julho de 2011-UFG. Goiânia: UFG; 2011 Available from: http://www.sbpcnet.org.br/livro/63ra/resumos/resumos/6155.htm

[20] Medeiros W, Torro-Alves N, Malloy-Diniz L, Minervino CM. Executive functions in children who experience bullying situations. Frontiers in Psychology. 2016;7:1197. DOI: 10.3389/fpsyg.2016.01197

[21] Burges PW, Simons JS. Theories of frontal lobe executive function: Clinical application. In: Halligan EPW, Wade DT, editors. Effectiveness of Rehabilitation for Cognitive Deficits. Oxford: Oxford University Press; 2005. pp. 211-232. DOI: 10.1093/acprof:oso/9780198526544.003.0018

[22] Diamond A. Executive functions. Annual Review of Psychology. 2013;**64**(135):68

[23] Malloy-Diniz LF, Sallum I, Fuentes D, Baroni LB, Costa DS, Paula JJ. In: Em LF, Malloy-Diniz D, Fuentes P, Mattos NA, editors. O exame das funções executivas, Avaliação Neuropsicológica. Porto Alegre: Artmed; 2018. pp. 90-105

[24] Uehara E, Charchat-Fichman H, Landeira-Fernandez J. Funções executivas: Um retrato integrativo dos principais modelos e teorias desse conceito. Revista Neuropsicologia Latinoamericana. 2013;**5**(3):25-37. DOI: 10.5579/rnl.2013.145

[25] Barkley RA. Problems with the concept of executive functioning. In: Barkley RA, editor. Executive Functions: What they Are, How they Work and Why they Evolved. New York: The Guilford Press; 2012. pp. 1-36

[26] Zelazzo PD, Cunningham WA. Executive function: Mechanisms underlying emotion regulation. In: Gross EJJ, editor. Handbook of Emotion Regulation. New York: The Guilford Press; 2007. pp. 135-158

[27] Zelazo PD, Müller U. Executive function in typical and atypical development. In: Goswami Em U, editor. Handbook of Childhood Cognitive Development. Blackwell: Minessota; 2002. pp. 445-469

[28] Norman DA, Shallice T. Action to action. In: Davidson ERJ, Schwartz GE, Shapiro D, editors. Consciousness and Self-Regulation. Boston: Springer; 1986. DOI: 10.1007/978-1-4757-0629-1

[29] Tirapu-Ustárroz J, García-Molina A, Luna-Lario B, Roig-Rovira T, Pelegrín-Valero C. Modelos de funciones y control ejecutivo. Revista de Neurologia. 2008;**46**(11):684-692

[30] De Bellis MD, Hooper SR, Spratt EG, Woolley DP. Neuropsychological findings in childhood neglect and their

relationships to pediatric PTSD. Journal of the International Neuropsychological Society. 2009;**15**:868-878. DOI: 10.1017/S1355617709990464

[31] Miyake A, Friedman NP, Emerson MJ, Witzki AH, Howerter A, Wager TD. The Unity and diversity of executive functions and their contributions to complex "frontal lobe" tasks: A latent variable analysis. Cognitive Psychology. 2000;**41**:49-100

[32] Baddeley AD, Hitch GJ. Working memory. In: Bower EGA, editor. Recent Advances in Learning and Motivation. New York: Academic Press; 1974. pp. 44-89

[33] Seabra AG, Reppold CT, Dias MD, Pedron AC. Modelo de funções executivas. In: Seabra EAG, Laros JA, Macedo EC, Abreu N, editors. Inteligência e funções executivas. Porto Alegre: Artmed; 2014. pp. 39-50

[34] Branco LD, Ponsoni A, Cotrena C. Funções executivas: definições, subcomponentes e bases neuroanatômicas. In: Zimmerman EN, Fonseca (Orgs.) RP, editors. Avaliação de linguagem e funções executivas em adultos. São Paulo: Memnon; 2017. pp. 13-23

[35] Wiebe SA, Espy KA, Charak D. Using confirmatory factor analysis to understand executive control in children: I. latent structure. Developmental Psychology. 2008;**44**(2):575-587

[36] Garon M, Bryson SE, Smith IM. Executive function in preschoolers: A review using an integrative framework. Psychological Bulletin. 2008;**134**(1):31-60. DOI: 10.1037/0033-2909.134.1.31

[37] Santos FH, Garcia RB, Piovezana ALRPD. O impacto da memória na aprendizagem e no desempenho acadêmico. In: Dias ENM, Mecca TP, editors. Avaliação Neuropsicológica cognitiva: Memória de trabalho. São Paulo: Memnon; 2019. pp. 32-42

[38] Alloway TP, Banner GE, Smith P. Working memory and cognitive styles in adolescents' attainment. British Journal of Educational Psychology. 2008;**80**(4):567-581

[39] Borges D, Dell'Aglio D. Funções cognitivas e Transtorno de Estresse Pós-Traumático (TEPT) em meninas vítimas de abuso sexual. Aletheia. 2009;**29**:88-102

[40] Cicchettia D, Handley ED. Child maltreatment and the development of substance use and disorder. Neurobiology of Stress. 2019;**10**:1-9. DOI: 10.1016/j.ynstr.2018.100144

[41] De Bellis MD, Morey RA, Nooner KB, Woolley DP, Haswell CC, Hooper SR. A pilot study of neurocognitive function and brain structures in adolescents with alcohol use disorders: Does maltreatment history matter? Child Maltreatment. 2019;**24**(4):374-388. DOI: 10.1177/1077559518810525

[42] Valentino K, Bridgett DJ, Hayden LC, Nuttall AK. Abuse, depressive symptoms, executive functioning, and overgeneral memory among a psychiatric sample of children and adolescents. Journal of Clinical Child & Adolescent Psychology. 2012;**41**(4):491-498. DOI: 10.1080/15374416.2012.660689

[43] Williams LCA, D'Affonseca SM, Correia TA, Albuquerque PP. Efeitos a longo prazo de victimization na escola. Revista Interinstitucional de psicologia. 2011;**4**(2):187

[44] den Kelder RP, Akker ALV, Geurst HM, Lindauer RJ, Overbeek G. Executive functions in trauma-exposed youth: A meta-analysis. European Journal of Psychotraumatology.

2018;**9**:1450595. DOI: 10.1080/20008198.2018.1450595

[45] Nooner KB, Hooper SR, De Bellis MD. An examination of sex differences on neurocognitive functioning and behavior problems in maltreated youth. Psychology Trauma. 2018;**10**(4):435-443. DOI: 10.1037/tra0000356

[46] Smith MK, Henry L, Messer D. Executive functioning: Developmental consequences on adolescents with histories of maltreatment. British Journal of Developmental Psychology. 2014;**32**:305-319

[47] Vasilevski V, Tucker A. Wide ranging cognitive deficits in adolescents following early life maltreatment. Neuropsychology. 2016;**13**(2):239-246

[48] Know Violence in Childhood. Ending Violence in Childhood. Global Report 2017. Know Violence in Childhood. New Delhi, India. Available from: https://resourcecentre.savethechildren.net/document/ending-violence-childhood-global-report-2017/

[49] Brancalhone PG, Fogo JC, Williams LCA. Crianças expostas à violência conjugal: avaliação do desempenho acadêmico. Psicologia: Teoria e Pesquisa. 2004;**20**(2):113-117

[50] Gathercole SE, Pickering SJ, Knight C, Stegmann Z. Working memory skills and educational attainment: Evidence from national curriculum assessments at 7 and 14 years of age. Cognitive Psychology. 2004;**18**(1):1-16. DOI: 10.1002/acp.934

[51] National Scientific Council on the Developing Child. The Science of Neglect: The Persistent Absence of Responsive Care Disrupts the Developing Brain: Working Paper No. 12. 2012. Available from: www.developingchild.harvard.edu